DANCING WITH
BROKEN BONES

Dancing with Broken Bones

Portraits of Death and Dying
Among Inner-City Poor

DAVID WENDELL MOLLER, Ph.D.

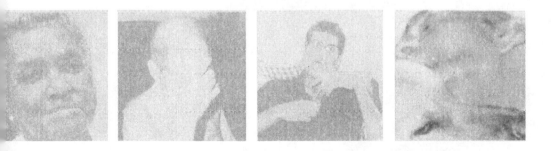

OXFORD
UNIVERSITY PRESS
2004

OXFORD
UNIVERSITY PRESS

Oxford   New York
Auckland   Bangkok   Buenos Aires   Cape Town   Chennai
Dar es Salaam   Delhi   Hong Kong   Istanbul   Karachi   Kolkata
Kuala Lumpur   Madrid   Melbourne   Mexico City   Mumbai
Nairobi   São Paulo   Shanghai   Taipei   Tokyo   Toronto

Published by Oxford University Press, Inc.
198 Madison Avenue, New York, New York, 10016
http://www.oup-usa.org

Oxford is a registered trademark of Oxford University Press

Library of Congress Cataloging-in-Publication Data
Moller, David Wendell.
Dancing with broken bones: portraits of death and dying among inner-city poor /
by David Wendell Moller.
p. cm.
ISBN 978-0-19-516534-0; 978-0-19-516526-5 (pbk.)
1. Urban poor—United States—Death—Case studies.
2. Terminal care—United States—Case studies.
3. Death—Social aspects—United States. I. Title.
HV4045.M65 2003   362.1'75'0869420973—dc21   2003042861

4 6 8 9 7 5
Printed in the United States of America
on acid-free paper

To

Greg Gramelspacher
Linda Kirchhoff
Jodi Groves
Mary Ciccarelli

In honor of the work you do and the persons you are.
I am blessed to have friends and colleagues such as these.

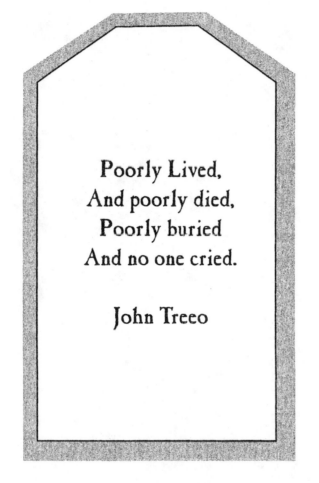

Poorly Lived,
And poorly died,
Poorly buried
And no one cried.

John Treeo

Pauper's gravestone as reported by Nathaniel Hawthorne.

PREFACE

A smile gently graced the face of Ernest as he lay dying. "I feel time is short. I'm getting close to the fence," he calmly remarked.

Ernest grew up in the Deep South. He was born in a cabin on November 28, 1917 in Stevenson, Alabama that had neither indoor plumbing nor electricity. Home birth was not unusual in the context of rural southern poverty at that time. In fact, home was the place where many in his community, including his siblings, came into this world. One practical result of not being born in a hospital was that a birth certificate was never issued to him. Neither was a Social Security number ever assigned. For most Americans, the idea of not having a birth certificate or Social Security number would be unfathomable, but for Ernest as a young boy in rural Alabama, it mattered little. These were merely bureaucratic documents that were inconsequential to his daily struggle to survive.

Throughout his youth, Ernest lived estranged from the economic and cultural mainstream. The struggle he and his family faced was real, and life was hard. His immense physical strength as a boy was an asset that enabled him to work long hours in the fields and survive the physical rigors of poverty. Being poor and black in the segregated South, however, was the curse of his birthright. He lived within a network of extended family for which poverty was not only a present reality but was both the past and future as well.

Seeking relief from economic and social hardship and in pursuit of a brighter future, he migrated north in 1932, winding up in New York City's Harlem. As a black man with exclusively agrarian-based survival skills, opportunities did not abound for Ernest. He survived the best he could, hustling and doing odd jobs. For eighteen months, his home was a corner newsstand, the day-old papers serving as his pillow and blanket. He reminisces about this time matter-of-factly and mostly without bitterness, yet his descriptions of the insufferable heat in the summer, how he would lie shivering during the cold of the winter, and the hardness of the concrete floor that served as his mattress and bed declare the degree of physical suffering he endured.

In the years that followed, he moved throughout the Midwest. Relationships with various girlfriends and wives resulted in nine children. Mental health problems led to violations of the law and subsequent incarcerations from which he ultimately escaped. His escape led to a life on the lam, a life he lived for more than three decades. He worked hard throughout these years, typically as a laborer and sometimes driving a cab. A false Social Security number was used to obtain employment and driver's licenses. In fact, in some of the union-based labor jobs he held Social Security taxes were withheld from his pay and presumably deposited into someone else's account. How he was able to get away with this deception for all those years is something we will never know.

During his time in Alabama, lacking identification meant nothing. For most of his adult life, through street savvy and skill, he was able to fudge and make due with false documents and a false identity, but all his success in deception came crashing down after being diagnosed with untreatable lung cancer. His physicians in the public hospital, where he was being treated as an "indigent patient," referred him to hospice after the diagnosis was made. Hospice immediately rejected him as a patient, however, because he was not enrolled in Medicare and they would not be reimbursed for their services. It seemed that the consequences of living marginalized and undocumented were finally catching up with him.

It was at this point that I first met Ernest. Linda, the social worker in the palliative care program at County Hospital, had heard about his situation and was on her way to make a home visit. She invited me along.

He was living in public housing with a friend who was a resident of the building. House rules allowed him to stay there two weeks, after which he would be required to move. In her initial assessment, Linda probed a bit about his family background, residential and work history, eligibility for various services, and what he understood about his illness. While initially evading most of her questions, he was straight forward in discussing his diagnosis and prognosis. "I have lung cancer, and they tell me it can't be treated," he stated, looking directly into her eyes. They talked for a while about how he was feeling and whether he was experiencing distressing symptoms or pain. Slowly the conversation returned to the seriousness of his illness, and he explained with ease and certainty that while he wanted to live as long as he could, death did not frighten him. "I see a mansion in the sky, and it is calling me," he said. "It has bright lights; it's up there," he noted while looking upward toward the heavens.

In the following days, Linda went to work on his most pressing problem: finding somewhere to live. This was not an easy task given his lack of income, insurance, and identification, but the director of a residence for homeless men discharged from the hospital stepped up to the plate. Mark provided a safe and comfortable place for Ernest to live, despite the fact that he was undocumented. Ernest integrated smoothly into his new environment. He was always glad to receive visitors. I would bring by medical students who were participating in a home-based educational program designed to unveil the stories and needs of inner-city dying poor. These visits were always appreciated, and he seemed to revel in his role as teacher to the next generation of physicians. Linda visited frequently, and they quickly became friends. As Ernest grew to trust her, he revealed much about life—its struggles, failures, and hopes. What mattered most to him at this point was salvation. He was fearful of going to hell as punishment for the imperfect way in which he lived.

As he grew sicker, and in particular because he was becoming incontinent, he was told that he would not be able to remain in this transitional residence much longer. A nursing home placement seemed to be the most appropriate option, but given his undocumented status, it would also be difficult to arrange. Linda, having anticipated the need weeks before, had been contacting nursing homes throughout the city. By dint of heroic effort, she was able to arrange for Ernest, as a charity case, to become a resident at the nursing home affiliated with County Hospital. This is where Ernest continues to live, having been there for the past five months.

Throughout his stay Ernest has yearned for social and spiritual connectedness. His pain and other troubling symptoms have been controlled remarkably well. From a physical standpoint, he has been generally comfortable, but his spiritual fears and sense of isolation, especially early on, have been sources of distress. In response, Barbara, the palliative care team chaplain, established a productive partnership with him. Along with a religiously devout volunteer, she worked energetically and successfully on self-forgiveness, stressing that "God has forgiven, now it is time for you to do the same." As a result of strong spiritual support, his fears of punishment have been quelled, and he is now able to face the end of his life with astonishing equanimity.

Linda continues to see him faithfully three times a week. He has grown to love her deeply, and she him. He waits urgently between visits for her to arrive and is always sad to see her go. "I pray for my friends every night, and it always brings a smile to my face," he says appreciatively.

Just this week he said to her, "I'm moving. Will you help me?" Asked to where he was moving, he replied, "Heaven." "Of course I will," she assured him. Thus, it would seem that a life that started out grimly, laced with poverty and racism, is ending peacefully in the nurturing arms of those who work by choice in a public hospital in service to the most vulnerable.

This brief snapshot illuminates some of the defining issues of a deeply hidden experience: dying while living within the confines of urban poverty. Coming to terms with dying is difficult enough. When poverty, alienation, and disempowerment surround the confrontation with mortality, suffering is often exacerbated and further hidden. Even though the general drift of our times is toward denial and avoidance of dying, there has been a splendid outpouring of recent writing wherein physicians, psychologists, mystics, and others have explored dying as an opportunity for growth and enlightenment. A common thread that ties much of this work together is how joys of discovery and fulfillment can emerge in the midst of struggle and suffering. While there is much that is important in these efforts to break the silence that surrounds death and dying in America, there is also an unintended bias toward chronicling the experience of those who are empowered. Many of these works discuss the ways individuals and families craft personalized responses to dying and death that involve creative and comforting expressions. Perhaps, as some have suggested, the baby boom generation, as it moves through the life cycle, is beginning to transform the ways Americans die. The same sense of empowerment and individualism that has served the boomers in life, it is speculated, is laying the foundation for transporting the ways of death into expressions that are both inwardly and outwardly creative. In this framework baby boomers are seeking creative responses to death that are consistent with the privileges of affluence and self-determination that have marked their lives. In fact, the recent series by Bill Moyers on the state of dying in America emphasized this phenomenon in its very title: On Our Own Terms. There are, however, individuals throughout society who do not possess the resources to shape and enact their deaths according to their own wishes, desires, and terms. Among these are people in the inner city whose lives have been shackled by poverty. These individuals frequently find themselves unable to assert control over dying. For them, anger, mistrust, and sadness prevail throughout the process. Lacking inspiration and revealing despair, their unsettling stories are typically ignored. In many ways the essence of their struggle in dying is defined by the struggle of having lived in poverty. Even when strength, resilience, and unbroken spirit govern the course of dying, the stories of the inner-city poor remain untold. Neglect in dying is therefore reflective of neglect in life, as the life stories of the poor usually remain unheard and unseen in the everyday flow of American life.

The purpose of this book is to give a voice and provide a face to their lives and suffering. In giving a voice to their sorrow, the injustice of poverty, the evil of racism, and the harm inflicted by inequality will be exposed. Its purpose is also to illustrate their uniqueness as persons in the hope that others will be better able to understand and respect their lives.

The material presented in Dancing with Broken Bones is the result of three research initiatives. The first, funded by the Open Society Institute, provided the opportunity to conduct extensive focus groups with patients, families, providers, and community members. The second, funded by the Indiana University Research Venture Fund, enabled a longitudinal study to be done. Patients were identified by staff physicians as having a life prognosis of twelve months or less. The doctors initially discussed the purpose of the project with patients. Those who expressed an initial willingness to participate received further details about the effort and the role they would play. After agreeing to participate, patients were followed throughout their illnesses to death. The third project was an elaboration of the second, whereby stories of patients and families were mined in longitudinal fashion, and student physicians were brought along to their homes for teaching purposes. The role of the students was to listen to the stories in the context of home and family so they could arrive at empathic understandings of how patients as persons are influenced by their economic and cultural backgrounds. This effort was made possible by the support of a grant from the Clarian Values Fund.

Those who participated consented to share their stories, having their narratives audiotaped and photos taken. Institutional Review Board consent for each of these related projects was obtained. Interactions with everyone who participated were loosely structured. The goal was to establish a relationship with individuals, following and observing them as they progressed through the process of dying. All conversations, whether in the home or elsewhere, were taped and transcribed in their entirety. Not only did I read the transcripts in writing this book, I listened to the tapes. Listening quietly to conversations that I had been part of, sometimes during chaotic circumstances, often provided a deepened understanding of their underlying feelings and experiences. Although some patients expressed a desire to have their real names used, all last names have been fictionalized.

Throughout this work I found that as relationships developed, trust blossomed. To a person, all who chose to participate continued to do so with enthusiasm, even gratitude. They were appreciative of the fact that others were interested in them and their stories. In allowing their experiences to be recorded and told, they chose to give a gift to others. A message I read in their eyes, all the more urgent for not being spoken, ran something like this: accept this gift not only with your minds and eyes as you read the narratives and look at the pictures, but with your hearts and souls as well. They hoped, I am sure, that in their dying they might be able to make a difference, perhaps thereby achieving a final triumph in a life during which they had been a matter of indifference to so many.

The stories you are about to read portray an invisible, complicated, and sometimes contradictory world. As the experiences of patients and families are revealed, the uniqueness of each individual will become apparent. Additionally, the portraits that emerge make vivid not just individual faces. They also reflect the moods, characters, and environments of the individuals. In this way, light is shed on both the internal and external world of the experience of dying in inner-city poverty. In extracting generalizations about the "invisible" experience of dying poor, some of which are hinted at in the brief vignette of Ernest with which I began, the following points can be made.

- Poverty inflicts substantial harm throughout life.
- Poverty exacerbates indignity and suffering throughout dying.

- Patients and families are often mistrustful and angry about care received.
- Patients are grateful for care received.
- Faith plays a prominent role in providing strength and resilience throughout dying.
- Social isolation intensifies suffering.
- Hidden and sometimes unexpected sources of strength and support emerge from family and community.
- The emergency room is often the front door to health care.
- The organization of care is frequently fragmented and lacks continuity.
- Funerals are extremely important rituals, and their cost creates enormous stress.

ACKNOWLEDGMENTS

This book would never have been possible without the support of others. There are many people to thank. Foremost are the individuals whose stories appear in the following pages. I am grateful to these patients. They have been the greatest teachers in my life, providing special memories and memorable moments. In many ways they became unique friends in their willingness to participate in a project that was so deeply personal. As unique relationships grew, they willingly and openly invited me into some very private parts of their lives. They were happy to know someone who showed an interest in them, and they wanted their stories to be told so others might benefit. They will always retain a very special place in my heart for their generosity, for their willingness to teach, and for making what began as a research initiative into a life-changing experience for me as a person and professional.

Greg Gramelspacher, David Smith, Betsy Fife, Dan Pesut, and Richard Gunderman helped form the project. Jenny Girod, who served as project manager, was a partner throughout much of the work. It is only her high sense of integrity that prohibits her name from appearing on the title page. The Division of Internal Medicine and Geriatrics at Indiana University School of Medicine and the Palliative Care Program at Wishard Health Services provided invaluable assistance and support. Special thanks go to Turkessa Earls for her patience and gentle ways. Monika Friend of the Indiana University School of Social Work and the Indiana University–Purdue University Indianapolis Department of Sociology provided invaluable editorial assistance along with an exacting attention to detail. Her technical expertise was a lifesaver for a disorganized technophobe and Luddite who still writes all his material on yellow legal pads.

For those unique individuals who work selflessly to serve the most vulnerable in the public hospital and to those who strive to bring humanism and empathy to the culture of medical education at Indiana University School of Medicine, I offer special acknowledgment of the work you do. Among them and their special qualities are

> Greg Gramelspacher, in recognition of his unassailable commitment to the poor
>
> Mary Ciccarelli, for the way she loves her patients
>
> Anne Zerr, for becoming a doctor's doctor in service to the poor
>
> Kathy and Gareth Gilkey, for their selfless devotion to others
>
> Jodi Groves, for her unparalleled skills in nursing and communication
>
> Meg Gaffney, in recognition of being the heart and conscience of Indiana University School of Medicine
>
> Gary Mitchell, for recognizing that the humanities are the hormones that drive the practice of medicine
>
> Linda Kirchhoff, for all she gives to others

Last but always first in my heart, I thank Binky for the love with which she has nurtured me for twenty-seven years.

It has been said that the poor will always be with us, yet despite their seemingly inevitable presence in American life, they are little understood. As an internal medicine resident remarked when making his first home visit to see a patient who was dying from Lou Gehrig's disease, "Even though I knew these neighborhoods existed, I never really knew these neighborhoods." A colleague added, "I will never think about the poor people in the same way again." In this spirit of transformation, as the stories and lives of the dying poor are revealed in *Dancing with Broken Bones*, I hope that others will come to the realization articulated years ago by Mother Teresa: "The poor, I do not tire of repeating this, are wonderful."

CONTENTS

DANCING WITH BROKEN BONES

Chapter

1

CROSSING THE TRACKS:
AN INTRODUCTION

Is name is Cowboy. The month is September, and Linda and I are on our way to visit him at home. However, this will be no ordinary visit, for Cowboy lives under a bridge in metropolitan Indianapolis. He is a striking, light-skinned seventy-three-year-old man of biracial descent. At first sight, he looks thin but vibrant. His marvelously bright eyes seem betrayed by an unclean appearance, and his weathered face reveals a life of long-term suffering and hardship. Greeting us with enthusiasm, he scurries inside and returns with gifts. He presents Linda with a bunch of freshly picked flowers. "I'm not going to tell you where I got them," he says to her mischievously. For me, he has a can of Pepsi wrapped in foil and accompanied with a straw. "You take this and drink it, it's good, you know," he instructs.

Immediately I sense that, although he lives in an unusual way, Cowboy is a unique and special man. He is engaging, articulate, and gracious. Despite these attractive qualities, however, he is rendered invisible, having been both disregarded and disdained by the thousands of people who literally travel over and past his home everyday. Daily he faces the challenges imposed by poverty, homelessness, mental illness, and recently diagnosed lung cancer, yet he remains fiercely independent, retaining great capacity for joy and love. Most people ignore, fear, or disrespect him because, in a culture of affluence and materialism, he embodies economic failure and moral shame. Nevertheless, his story, all the more urgent because it is typically not told, contains important lessons about societal responsibility, empathetic connection, the nature of suffering, and the possibilities for transcendence.

1

Cowboy has lived here for years. The site once housed a colony of homeless men, but they were all chased away by the police. Cowboy was allowed to stay because of his respectful demeanor and the fact that he was judged not to be a threat or a nuisance. He loves his home and speaks affectionately about it, calling it "the cave." He is keen on giving us a tour of the premises.

"This is the lounge area," he begins, referring to the first section we come upon after passing through the plastic tarp that serves as the front door. Two bar stools are placed against the back wall, both covered with a film of soot. Remarkably, in this dirty and dingy place that Cowboy calls home, an ironic sense of order and neatness is evident. All his personal items, from medicines, razors, and shave cream to soaps, deodorant, and toiletries, are impeccably organized. He knows where his every possession is and takes pride in telling us that he is always fixing things up. "I'm an organizer and fixer," he says with a wry laugh. "Always have been."

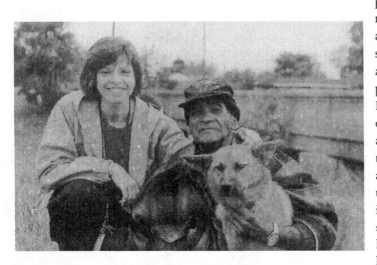

Linda on a home visit with Cowboy and Cowgirl.

Continuing with the tour, he takes us deeper into the cave, apologizing for the lack of light. "My gas lantern is broken but it'll be fixed soon. So when you come back, things will be nicer." This area is past a dead tree that we have to climb around or under and contains all kinds of paraphernalia one might expect a homeless person to have: shopping cart, charcoal grill in which wood is burned for heat, boxes of clothes, and torches filled with a mixture of diesel fuel and gasoline to provide a bit of lighting. Smoke from the burning fire fills the air, and I cannot help but think it is no wonder he is dying from lung cancer. Venturing deeper still into the furthest and darkest recesses of the cave, we come to the bedroom. Here is a twin-size box spring and mattress that has sheets, two blankets, and pillows. There are more boxes of clothes against the wall. Next to the bed is a table where he keeps things he might want during the night. Immediately behind his bed is "the toilet." This is a cardboard box that he fills with dirt, "You know, like cat's litter," he unashamedly explains. "I empty it everyday, but usually I go to the bathroom out in the neighborhood." Somehow, I feel impressed with

Cowboy's serenity in living with poverty.

I later discovered poverty has been the only life he has ever known. Cowboy grew up in the Deep South, picking cotton on a plantation. "We were *beyond poverty*," he lamented. "Our 'boss man' would lend us enough money to get through the month, but it always ran out in the third or fourth week. We were always

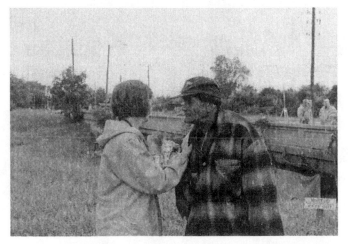

Outside the cave receiving gifts of flowers and Pepsi.

in debt to him and could never get out of it." In a very strange way, the foundation for self-sufficiency that would enable him to live productively as an urban, homeless person was laid in the impoverishment of his youth. As his family literally struggled to eat and survive, Marvin, as he was named at birth, learned the arts of hustling and entrepreneurship. He raised some chickens that provided eggs and meat, along with a small monthly income. "And I'm not going to tell you how I got it all started," he would tease. He did odd jobs for affluent families and earned enough money to eat well

throughout the month. "They would go hungry, but not me," he often said with a trace of bitterness in his voice, referring to his family. His memories of those days in Mississippi are mixed. He takes enormous pride in having survived, especially in his ability to find ways of exceeding the standard of living to which others in his family and

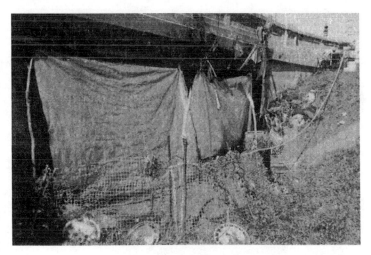

The outside of the cave was decorated with flags on September 11, 2001.

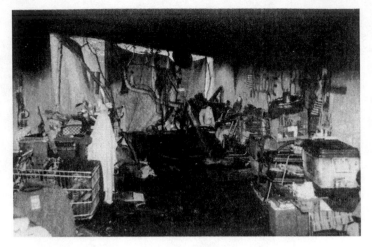

Inside the cave.

community suc-
cumbed. Even so,
the circumstances of
economic impover-
ishment created enor-
mous hardship that
became his constant
companion and de-
fined the boundaries
of his life.

In addition to the
injuries inflicted by
severe poverty, prej-
udice and racism also
shaped his youthful
experiences. Born
out of wedlock, he
was conceived by a mother of African-American heritage, while his father was
Greek. Even before his birth his mother was sharply ridiculed by her family and community. She suffered this rejection less for having become pregnant outside of marriage at the age of fourteen than because her baby's father was of a different race. As
a result of his conception and birth, life was made difficult for Marvin's mother, and
she deeply resented him. She abused him physically and verbally. He was another
mouth to feed, and his presence in her community was a constant source of insult and
derision.

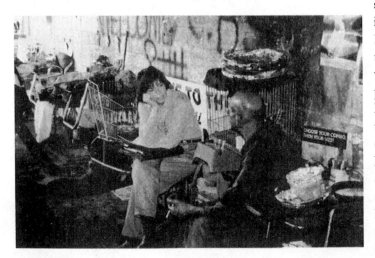

A social work assessment.

For thirteen years
she passed on this
iniquity to her son.
He angrily explains
that those years
were filled with
physical and verbal
harm: how boiling
water was poured
over him, the scars
being visible still to-
day; that his mother
and cousins would
beat him regularly;
that he was repeat-
edly called the most
vicious names by his

family and neighbors; and that he was told on more than one occasion that "everybody would be better off if you were dead." Cowboy's boyhood experiences torment him to this day. He speaks with rage and fury every time he mentions his mother. Her words "I wish I had flushed you down the toilet" remain a hurtful mantra that he has never been able to reconcile. Just as regrettable, Cowboy has passed the legacy of harm on to his own children. He has three by different women. One child is a Christian pastor. Another graduated from Harvard but went on to sell bootleg goods out of the back of his van. The third, his only daughter, is in middle-level management for a national pharmaceutical company. The children want absolutely nothing to do with their father, and Cowboy despises them. "They just don't accept my lifestyle," he says with resentment. Both Linda and I have sought his permission to contact the children so they may say goodbye to their dying father

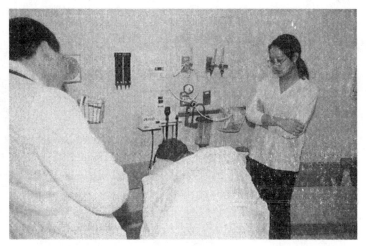

Shivering from hypothermia and pneumonia in the emergency room.

and attend his funeral. He becomes irate every time the matter is brought up, and we have been instructed never to mention it again. I cannot help but contemplate how the injustice of poverty and the wickedness of racism, which Marvin suffered as a boy, have influenced not only his view of the world but his capacity to relate to it. I often ponder what his life would have been like had not the severity of poverty and evil of prejudice overwhelmed his body and soul during his formative years.

When he was thirteen, his mother, wanting to be entirely rid of her burden, sent him to Indianapolis to live with a grandmother. Although he yearned for an education in his new environment, he was told he was too stupid to learn and should accept who he was, so he turned to the streets and received an education of a different sort. He joined the army during the Korean era at the age of eighteen and served for two years in Texas. After being honorably discharged, he worked at many jobs, including driving taxis, bartending, and shining shoes. He always took great delight in "dressing fine and enjoying life." With money in his pocket, he dressed to impress the

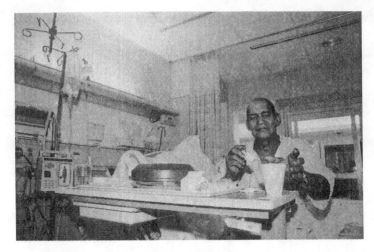

Having been stabilized with antibiotics, Cowboy enjoys a meal in the progressive intensive care unit.

ladies, referring to this self-presentation as "cash and flash-flash and cash." He loved and still is passionate about music, which he describes as "my true mistress." Nonetheless, throughout his life he was always haunted by a sense of exile, never feeling comfortable with himself regardless of his surroundings. His upbringing coupled with his failed marriages and other failed relationships has created pain and mistrust, both of which have increasingly become manifest in mental pathology. He does not have a formal diagnosis. However, the best informal medical opinion is that he is manic and perhaps mildly schizophrenic.

Recently, Cowboy had been having enormous difficulty breathing, and his legs had swollen elephantinelike. He rode his bicycle to the local public hospital and was found wandering the hallways. He was immediately taken to the emergency room (ER), where he was evaluated and subsequently admitted to the hospital. Tests revealed that he had lung cancer. After being stabilized and regaining some strength, he would sneak out in the afternoons. The staff assumed he was just running back to the streets for illicit purposes, but these afternoon disappearances had a different objective. He was

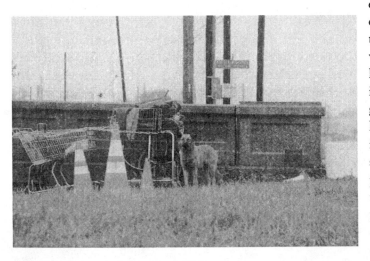

Cowgirl keeps watch for the return of Cowboy.

returning to the cave to feed Cowgirl. "She's my best friend and I have to take care of her," he said about his nine-month-old puppy.

Since his diagnosis, Cowboy's life has increasingly become connected to the public hospital system. He began chemotherapy, has met the palliative care team, has spoken to medical students, and has been to the ER four times. Each trip to the ER resulted in admission to the progressive intensive care unit (PICU). His experience as a patient in a public hospital has been both positive and negative. He loves visits by medical students, who have taken an interest in this man from "the other side of the tracks." He thinks the world of his oncologist, although he has met her only once. He loves Linda, the palliative care social worker, and cannot wait for "Dr. G.," the medical director, to visit. On the other hand, he has been the recipient of some abusive and impatient treatment by some nurses in the ER, who have been frustrated by his return visits. (He had not been fully compliant in taking the antibiotics to treat his pneumonia.) He was

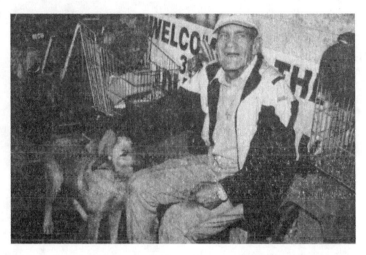

A joyful welcome home and reunion. "She's my best friend," he quips.

confused and disorderly during his last PICU admission, and the nurses exacerbated the situation by huddling outside his door, trying to figure out how to deal with him. He overheard the muddled tones of their conversation and became paranoid because they were talking about him. He started snarling at them, and they decided it was necessary for him to be restrained.

Fortunately, at this time Linda was stopping by for a visit. She was able to instruct the nurses about Cowboy's history and needs. Although his history is indeed complex, his needs are rather simple. He needs to know that he and his suffering matter, he needs reassurance that he will not be abandoned, and he requires recognition and respect for his uniqueness as a person. Linda went into his room. Sitting on his bed, she took his hand and spoke with a comforting tone. Within a matter of minutes, the transformation was phenomenal. His ranting and raving were replaced by calm and gratitude. Having witnessed such a remarkable change in behavior, the

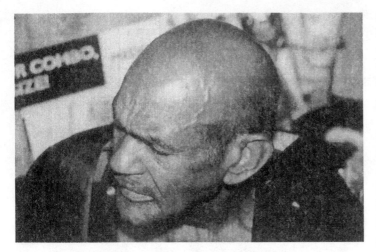

Painful reminiscence of poverty and prejudice in the Deep South.

nurses learned how better to interact with Cowboy, and their relationship with him has improved significantly.

Cowboy was discharged from this hospital admission early in November. He is currently living in a room at the local YMCA. The rent has been paid for two weeks by a Catholic layperson who runs a metropolitanwide street ministry. Cowboy goes each day to the cave to check on Cowgirl. His faith in God is a source of strength during this difficult time.

"I'm surprised you ask me about God," he admonished when I questioned him about his beliefs. "God makes all this possible. Yup, he does," he said with conviction. I noticed out of the corner of my eye a Bible neatly placed on a table.

"I don't read it so much anymore, and the ministers, they have rejected me a long time ago," he adds. I find it interesting that his faith is as private as it is deep.

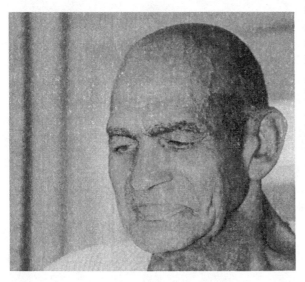

Speaking about how "God makes all things possible" brings comfort and a smile.

His belief is strong, but his disconnection from a faith community and its supportive rituals seem intractably solidified by his lifestyle and its rejection by local churches. Sadly, the cave is located within 500 feet of a church, whose clergy and members have no involvement whatsoever with Cowboy. The result of this separation is that he is facing the end of life with regrettable spiritual isolation.

I do not know what the future holds for him. He could die this week or live for six months. It is also unclear where he will live after his two weeks at the YMCA are over. Winter is coming, he is sick, and something will have to be worked out for him, and hopefully for Cowgirl as well.

This book, like the example with which I began, is about a most profound experience: living with dying while living in poverty. When we contemplate the experience of dying in American culture, there is much that indicates that dying and its related sufferings are plunged deep beneath the surface of cultural interest and concern. The facts of dying—pain, weakness, incontinence, soiled sheets, loss of bodily function, emotional anguish, and exhaustion— are noticeably absent from the prevailing images and experiences of our daily lives. We live in a culture in which relationships with dying persons are reserved for professionals who provide necessary services. A few intimates, out of duty or devotion, may accompany loved ones into their deaths. The rest of the community, in-

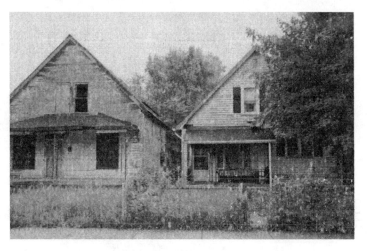

Crossing the tracks.

cluding friends and neighbors, are not likely to be connected in any meaningful way to the sufferings of dying others. Disgust, fear, individualism, disinterest, and busyness are some of the reasons that underlie the widespread aversion to associating with dying persons. As a result, the experience of dying and the difficulties that surround it are hidden almost to the point of invisibility.

The world of the inner-city poor is similarly hidden. When viewed from the perspective of most of us, the inner-city poor live in a feared netherland of filthy streets and unsafe neighborhoods filled with drugs, violence, and dilapidated housing. Our perception of the life they lead in these decaying conditions is equally forlorn and fearful. Undoubtedly, when we think of the inner-city poor, we envision lives and homes tattered by alcohol, violence, financial urgency, personal irresponsibility, and dysfunctional behavior. This world of turmoil and disorder is both frightening and foreign. It is a struggle for even those most compassionate and enlightened to understand what it means to live in these circumstances. As a result, we tend to think little of the inner-city poor and what it must mean to face daily the challenges of poverty. Although we might listen to news reports about the suffering of the poor and catch a glimpse of their lives as we drive through "bad neighborhoods," we ultimately give little thought to them.

Decades ago Michael Harrington wrote that the poor, ever with us, tend to become increasingly invisible. Ralph Ellison echoed a similar theme in his chilling portrayal of the invisibility of the black man in the inner city. As I formed relationships with patients and families in this project, I sought to penetrate this invisibility. Venturing "across the tracks," I entered into lives that were unfamiliar to me, both personally and professionally. The specific goal was to journey to that especially unspoken and alien place where suffering, dying, and death intersect with poverty. At this junction I found deep crises and human misery—both of which were intensified because of "double invisibility": the poor are shunned because they are the economic and social failures in affluent America; the dying are shunned because, in a culture of denial, the experience of dying has become fraught with meaninglessness and fear. Thus, in a society of abundance and optimism about the future, the dying poor are the quintessential violators of the American dream: they live in the shame of poverty and with the unpleasantness of dying.

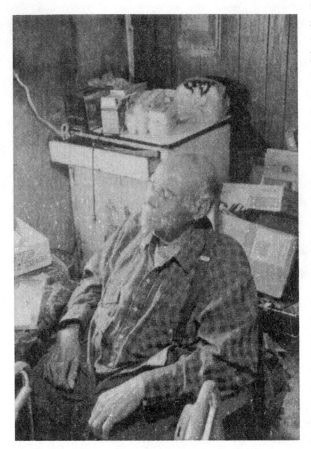

Jesse at home in the house he built forty-one years earlier.

Even so, I also discovered something unexpected. While set apart from mainstream culture, the "invisible" neighborhoods of the inner-city poor are home to individuals and families who display enormous spirit and courage at life's most difficult time. In meaningful ways their lives are filled with resilience, unspoken spirit, and optimism. For example, to the outsider, Jesse's living conditions were dingy, dirty, and malodorous. For Jesse, however, this was his beloved home. Goats roamed his yard. To the outsider they were a source of ridicule. For Jesse, they provided daily milk. It is no wonder that he resisted the idea of moving to a nursing home. "I've lived here for forty-one years, and I don't want to leave," he said with an engaging smile. Thus, in viewing Jesse from the outside, it might be easy to judge his living situation as deplorable, but in getting to know him in his world, it became clear why he felt comfortable and content in the home he personally built.

In an important sense, then, the spirit of the dying poor remains unseen. They have been cast off and dispossessed by a culture distracted by other interests. They have no face and little voice. This book is about providing a face and offering a voice to speak on their behalf. The conversations in which we engaged facilitated understanding and empathy, which in turn allowed me to establish some powerful and intimate relationships with individuals and their families. In fact, what began as an intellectually crafted research project ultimately became a life-changing experience. In immeasurable ways I am thankful to these patients and families for deepening my insights, broadening my knowledge, and enriching my life. I have also gained a deep respect for the courage it took for them to allow me to enter their lives during such a difficult time. They thought often of you (the people to whom I would tell their story), I am sure, and wondered how they would be perceived when they did not look or feel their best. They worried a little bit about how they would be represented but trusted that I would serve them well. The responsibility is huge; I must share their stories in a way that honors their lives and deaths. Thus, while this book is about themes and issues that stem from the interconnections among class, status, race, and dying, it is foremost about people. When ideas, themes, and scholarly analysis enter, they do so only because they are directly relevant to the lives, sufferings, and deaths of real people.

Perhaps the crowning indignity of a life lived in poverty about which no one cares is a death died in poverty while the culture smiles indifferently. The epitaph that begins this book was observed on a gravestone by Nathaniel Hawthorne in Lillington Churchyard, near Lexington Spa, England. As Hawthorne writes, the words are a fitting testimonial to a forlorn existence of living and dying in poverty while disinterest and disdain are the prevailing sentiments of the surrounding community.

> It would be hard to compress the story of a cold and luckless life, death, and burial into fewer words, or more impressive ones; at least, we found them impressive, perhaps because we had to recreate the inscription by scraping away the lichens from the faintly-traced letters. The grave was on the shady and damp side of the church, endwise towards it, the head-stone being within about three feet of the foundation-wall; so that, unless the poor man was a dwarf, he must have been doubled up to fit him into his final resting place. No wonder that his epitaph murmured against so poor a burial as this! His name, as well as I could make it out, was Treeo—John Treeo, I think—and he died in 1810, at the age of seventy-four. The gravestone is so over-grown with grass and weeds, so

covered with unsightly lichens, and so crumbly with time and foul weather, that it is questionable whether anybody will ever be at the trouble of deciphering it again. But there is a quaint and sad kind of enjoyment in defeating (to such slight degree as my pen may do it) the probabilities of oblivion for poor John Treeo and asking a little sympathy for him, half a century after his death.

Unfortunately, many people still die in a lonely and separated state, their isolation and stigma worsened by being poor in a culture of affluence. This probably should not be a matter of astonishment in a society that thinks little about the human misery of living and dying in poverty. In fact, dying in poverty is more likely an occurrence of little social consequence precisely because we live in a society that hardly thinks about these issues.

The consequences of widespread societal indifference are, however, deeply felt by many of the dying poor and their loved ones. Perhaps there are no more persuasive words to express this than those of Mr. Wheeler, who was dying from stomach cancer. His cancer had been diagnosed extremely late largely because, despite working all of his life, he was health care uninsured and used the ER of the county hospital as his primary "doctor's office." Notice a striking similarity between Hawthorne's description of John Treeo and the despairing words of Mr. Wheeler:

We have been cast aside, disregarded, and forgotten about.

This book is part of a commitment to making sure that the lives and deaths of the patients whose stories enrich these pages never sink into oblivion. The degree to which I succeed is a testament to the richness and dignity of their lives. The degree to which I do not is a reflection of my own omissions and failures. I hope that as you get to know these courageous individuals, you will come to appreciate the unique difficulties they faced in their struggles to live with dying within the grip of urban poverty.

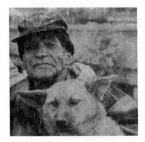

Chapter

2

DYING POOR:
AN INVISIBLE WORLD

I begin with a description of some of the life issues that affect particular individuals in order to bring the human experience of dying poor into focus. As you come to know them, you will notice that in their unique ways they suffered deeply. They lived within an inescapable complex of terrors: the nagging fear of death, the pain of bodily deterioration, and the eerie isolation that comes from realizing that "finally their time had arrived." These terrors were often compounded by a sense of alienation, medical uncertainty, poverty, family fragmentation, and mistrust. To a person, however, despite individual variations, these individuals displayed a surprising strength in getting used to the idea of dying. Their lifetime experiences with poverty blended together ironically with their newly found encounter with mortality. From the onset I was struck by their absence of bitterness about having lived their lives in poverty. This is not to suggest that these individuals did not feel the sting of poverty and its life-limiting impositions. Instead, they understood poverty as a cross to bear. As a result, they did not obsess about its deleterious consequences for the quality of their lives. Rather, despite enormous suffering that was often fueled by chaos, anger, and suspicion, they usually endured their illnesses similarly: with a graceful dignity and inner strength. As one person who had recently been told that he had rapidly spreading lung cancer and less than a year to live said:

> I know I'm not going to make it. Fifty-one is young to die, but with
> so much violence and destruction in the streets, many never make
> it that far. I'm grateful that I have.

Another expressed this sentiment of acceptance and gratitude with astonishing simplicity:

I'm still living and not complaining.

This attitude of equanimity may seem odd in a culture that fears dying so much as ours. Nonetheless, despite widespread suffering and bodily destruction, there was seldom an impression of urgency in their confrontations with dying. In fact, a startling gratitude was expressed by more than a few, rooted in faith in God and relationships with others. These individuals were typically deeply faithful and fully assured that the mystery of death would be revealed with beautiful result—not by machines, or science, or doctors, or medications, but by God. Their joy may have been muted by the harsh physical and emotional realities of dying. Nevertheless, they faced their personal extinction with unfettered confidence that God was with them. For most of these dying persons and their loved ones, God provided a sweetness, comfort, and security to their lives that otherwise would not have been possible given the incessant demands of living in inner-city poverty. The promise of peace and heaven was unparalleled in importance as they faced the reality of dying, even to those few whose faith had been less strong throughout their lives.

Relationships were also extremely important in their lives. They needed to know that their lives, suffering, and deaths mattered. They were deeply grateful to loved ones who provided support. Their need for connectedness while dying was deep, so much so that sometimes they idealized the role significant others played in their lives. They also worried about how their loved ones would fare in their absence and yearned to reconcile differences when they existed. Mrs. Angel, for example, emphasized how important family connections are and how they are made more urgent by the approach of death. Her description of the final Christmas with her dying husband, a Christmas made all the more special because it would be their last together, reveals a spirit and inner strength:

I love Christmas. . . . I put up a tree the year my husband died in April. He was able to help me decorate it. He always did the lights around the house and windows, decorate the tree and everything. And this year he was so sick, but he made himself. I think he forced himself—pushed himself to make it until that Christmas, and make it a good Christmas. Because I think in a way he knew it was to be his last Christmas, and it was a good Christmas in spite of that fact. The whole family was here. You know he could handle these daughters of mine better than I ever will . . . Yes, he could. It was a good Christmas despite the fact that he was dying. Yes. It was good because I could see he always loved Christmas and Thanksgiving. Those were good days. He said, "Oh, Mama would just fix big meals and everything." He loved the holidays. He would just go all out, dec-

orating the house and the tree, buying presents for everybody, taking
pictures. He just loved the holidays. . . . I do too, and it was a good
Christmas. I knew it would be his last. He knew it would be his last
and we made the best of it, the best we could, you know.

Relationships and the memories they engendered were deeply cherished. They offered comfort in the face of sadness and strength in the face of loss. In fact, despite
the existence of chaos, some family dysfunction, and neglect, many of the inner-
city poor I came to know were rich in the presence of some special caring relationships that supported them into their deaths.

Lest I overidealize the experiences of the inner-city poor at the end of life, I has-
ten to add that enormous difficulty and suffering filled their lives. In the inner-city
public hospital, where ninety-four percent of the patients do not have private
health care insurance, poverty significantly shaped the experience of dying and the
care that was rendered. In this regard, poverty mattered in the homes and communities where the patients lived and died as well as in the hospitals, clinics, and nursing homes in which they received care.

First and foremost, dying in the network of services provided by the public hospital is not a matter of choice. Poor dying persons wind up there because no other
hospital will take them. The typical entry into the public hospital system for poor
persons is captured effectively in the following:

> I moved to Indianapolis, and I got sick with pneumonia. An ambu-
> lance took me to one hospital and they transferred me to County.
> They got me on a program out there—the indigent program.

It can hardly be debated that "dying on their own terms" is severely restricted for
America's poor. Financial circumstance limits their options to choose between and
among services. Interestingly, for some the lack of choice hardly mattered because
they felt so deep a sense of appreciation for the care they received. For others it
mattered a lot, and these patients often complained bitterly about the care they received. Of those who were appreciative, many felt a strong sense of allegiance and
connection to the institution and its caregivers:

> It's like my second home because they do so much for me.

Another adds:

> We took cases of Pepsi to the staff because they were excellent.

The words of Annie, an eighty-year-old woman who was dying in Deerfield
Village (County's nursing home), also echoes this theme of thankfulness:

> You know that for the past months I have not been able to take care
> of myself. I am grateful to the people who take care of me here.

Perhaps the strong sense of loyalty that some feel toward "their hospital" is best captured by the following:

> I wouldn't go anywhere else.

Contrasting with this spirit of gratitude were others who expressed significant discontent with the experience of living with dying within the public hospital health system. Their complaints revolved around common themes of undignified treatment, lack of respect, the belief that they received inferior care because they were poor, and a reluctance to trust their providers. The inner-city poor, especially African Americans, are sometimes suspicious of the intentions of their physicians. These issues of mistrust typically originate elsewhere, such as from the legacy of Tuskegee, a preformed wariness of authority figures spawned by the experiences of a life lived in poverty, feeling intellectually and personally alienated from their doctors, and so on. For example, one Friday morning the medical director and social worker of County's palliative care team made a home visit to a man who had colon cancer. The man, who was extremely sick, was experiencing gastrointestinal distress and bowel obstruction. The team entered a walkup building that had just that week been condemned. The electricity was scheduled to be turned off sometime that day, and the resident had no plans for replacement housing. In fact, he was planning simply to continue living there without electricity until he was forcibly removed. On entering it was impossible not to notice the squalid conditions. Walls were cracked, the carpet was tattered and dirty, the atmosphere was unpleasant, dirty dishes overflowed from the sink, and an unmistakable odor of feces dominated the air. Throughout the home visit the patient, a sixty-seven-year-old African-American male, was resisting the efforts of the physician to prescribe a gastrointestinal procedure that would help ease some of his abdominal and bowel symptoms. In fact, the patient kept arguing with the physician, adamantly stating, "I don't have an obstruction." The physician responded, "Yes, you do, my friend." The patient curtly retorted, "How do you know?" The patient, Mr. Mellon, was unwilling to accept the physician's account of the medical facts and kept resisting the proposed plan of treatment. The social worker, correctly sensing that Mr. Mellon was having a difficult time accepting his diagnosis, emphathetically discussed with him how difficult it is to get used to the idea of having such a serious illness. The conversation was much appreciated by Mr. Mellon, and the social worker, recognizing that she had made a connection with the patient, skillfully brought the discussion back to his treatment options. In this conversation she asked Mr. Mellon directly "Mr. Mellon, do you trust Dr. G.?" He unflinchingly responded "No."

Any objective observer would have agreed that the care Mr. Mellon was receiving was extraordinary. The team willingly traveled to his residence. Comfortably, and without judgment, they entered into the foul and dingy living conditions. They compassionately listened to him and passionately presented a plan that would address his medical and social needs. Despite the exemplary caring behaviors of the team, Mr. Mellon was reluctant to believe two things: (*1*) that he was as sick as he was and (*2*) that he could actually trust this doctor who lived in a world about which Mr. Mellon was already suspicious.

Issues of mistrust often were connected to a distinct belief among patients that they were inadequately served by the public hospital. For example, Mr. Iris, himself a double kidney transplant patient, complained regularly about the different treatment he felt his wife, who was dying of lung cancer, received at County compared to the care she received when she was referred to University Hospital, where most patients have private health-care insurance. He also complained that the doctors and nurses at County disrespected his role as a caring participant in his wife's illness and often were impatient with and unresponsive to his questions. His belief, strong and straightforward, that poor patients receive inferior care at the public hospital was expressed in the following words:

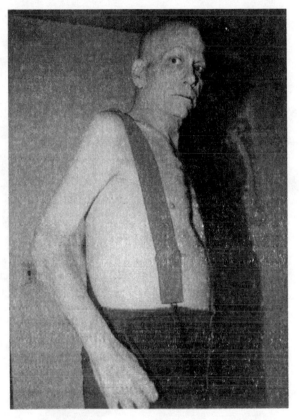

"We have been cast aside, disregarded, and forgotten about," remarked an angry Bill Wheeler.

We get treated differently at County because we are poor.

Mr. Wheeler, a man in his mid-fifties who was dying from stomach cancer, also spoke bitterly about the care he received at County. In fact, he was eagerly looking forward to becoming eligible for Medicare so he could choose another venue in which to receive health-care services. When asked at what hospital he liked to get his care, he responded:

It doesn't matter, just as long as it is not at County.

Mr. White, whom I will discuss in greater depth later, was also very bitter. His resentment was directed toward the care he and his wife received in Deerfield Village. At the age of seventy-two, he had been diagnosed with esophageal cancer and had decided not to be treated with chemotherapy. He was the primary caretaker of his wife of forty-three years, who herself was sick. Recognizing that he would soon be unable to take adequate care of his beloved wife, Mr. White decided that going to the nursing home would be best for him and his wife. Initially, he was grateful. The arrangements for admission to Deerfield Village were made quickly and with little imposition on them. His prized possessions, a console color television and a comfortable reclining chair, were moved from their home into their room. Most important, he was spared the increasingly impossible task of taking care of his wife. After a week or so, however, he became increasingly dissatisfied with the care they both were receiving. His complaints ranged from meals not being delivered or being delivered late, to a perception that the staff held a negative attitude toward them, to a bitter grumbling about how his wife's toileting and bathing needs were being neglected. Unlike Annie, who died thankful for the

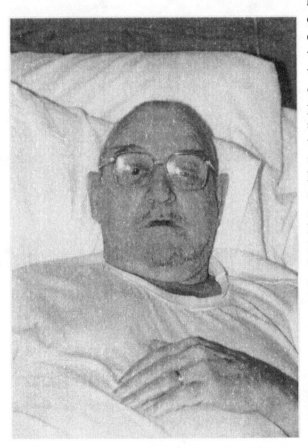

"It happened again. This time she lay in her own shit for seven hours," Mr. White bemoaned.

care she received, Mr. White lived and died at Deerfield Village bitter and sad. His bitterness is fully revealed by the caption that underscores the picture on the preceeding page.

Perhaps even more poignant than the anger and disappointment of dissatisfied patients is the absence of resentment on the part of those who have every reason to be upset with the care they receive. It is fair to suggest that, for some, this lack of assertiveness and anger has its roots deep within the experience of poverty. Living everyday with the chaos, stress, and indignity of inner-city poverty creates, for many, a level of tolerance that most of us would find impossible. In this regard, it is not unusual for patients to accept care with which they are unhappy because they have accepted a lifetime of economic and social indignities about which they are unhappy. In a strange sense, many patients often felt their suffering in the face of disease was just "one more bad thing to endure." Thus, despite many variations in form and meaning, disease and dying are often borne with a sense of equanimity that flows from the constant adjustments required by a life lived in poverty.

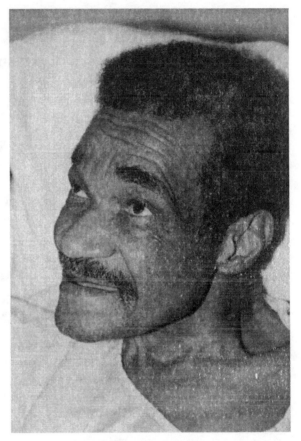

"It's okay. I can deal with this," remarks J. W.

This absence of bitterness, even when it should perhaps be forthcoming, is illustrated in the story of J. W. Green. Mr. Green was a sixty-year-old man whose prostate cancer was spreading throughout his spine. As the disease attacked his central nervous system, he was at the threshold of becoming a quadriplegic. Day after day he would lie on his back, unable to move in his bed in the nursing home. Hideous bedsores developed on his bottom. They were painful, infected, and smelled horrible. Mr. Green developed these sores because the nursing home staff did not move or turn him with any consistency. Despite the fact that he suffered great physical and personal indignity, he remained uncomplaining throughout the ordeal. Remarkably, throughout his dying, despite great worry about isolation and abandonment, he achieved great calm. In large part because of his unwavering faith in God, he was even able to experience moments of joy.

It should also be noted that, for the most part, those patients who were clearly angry, such as Mr. Wheeler and Mr. White, seldom, if ever, expressed their dissatisfaction directly to their care providers. While many patients, regardless of social or economic status, struggle to assert themselves directly to physicians, the situation for the dying poor is different. In all fairness, their passivity must be understood within the context of having lived a life in poverty, and continually having had to deal with an onslaught of social and economic degradation. In the constancy of poverty, little could be done to affect the circumstances of their lives. So they typically submitted to its harshness and indignities, although sometimes in destructive ways. This attitude of submission seemed to carry over to accepting indignities of care that more affluent and empowered individuals would never tolerate.

Thus, in our culture in which dying and suffering have become taboo, it is correct to say that most dying patients, independent of economic status, are disarmed and vulnerable. In their vulnerability it is understandable that many may not fully act in an empowered and assertive manner, especially when they are so dependent on the authority and skills of their physicians. However, the dying poor, who are especially vulnerable, often experience far greater feelings of disempowerment. This disempowerment was frequently expressed in a variety of discordant attitudes and behaviors on the part of patients. Sometimes it manifested itself in personal and family disorder. The crucial point is, however, that the chaos associated with the experience of dying poor in the inner city is tethered to the experience of having lived in poverty in urban America.

Clearly, it must be said, the American experience of living in poverty is not the same as is that for impoverished persons in developing nations. There, the daily struggle is to avoid starvation and death. In America poverty is more about the relative absence of money. Nonetheless, poverty in America ferociously attacks the bodies and souls of individuals, families, and communities. In many ways American poverty is as much about social experience as financial deprivation. Thus, although the financial circumstances of the poor in America may not lead directly to the threat of dying from starvation, we know that the poor suffer disproportionate incidences of disease and mortality. They endure deeper despair, higher levels of depression, and greater injury to mental health. They also experience and suffer social stigma and rejection directly related to being poor in a culture of affluence.

It is no secret that money and materialistic display are driving forces of cultural life. "Lifestyles of the rich and famous" have always fascinated the American people, and monetary success is a cherished value. As a culture, we long for financial success, often judging friends, neighbors, strangers, and ourselves by it. In this equation human worth is filtered through the lens of materialistic success. More is better. Ownership is a sacred value that perpetuates itself by cultivating a love of things. Money is treasured not only because it can bring peace, security, and joy to life but also because it grows the portfolio. Again, more is better, and tremendous energy goes into producing, consuming, and displaying possessions. Thus, in many ways material success is the cornerstone of the American way of life. We desire it deeply and evaluate the worth of others and ourselves by it.

Although we might be envious of others who have achieved material success, we are also voyeuristically obsessed with peeping into their lives. Our fascination with celebrities and the associated prevalence of tabloid journalism demonstrate our strong cultural preoccupation with social and economic status. In the entertainment and sports industries, for example, the media manufacture celebrities, and their public stature is supported by the thirst of the American public for a connection to their lives, no matter how superficial. In this context, money dominates: it creates celebrity, and celebrity earns more of it.

Far removed from this world, the poor are truly on "the other side of the tracks," both economically and socially. The context of financial want that defines their lives not only creates hardships in daily living but also elicits the moral judgment of others. Frankly, the ugly and simple truth is that the human and social worth of the poor is denigrated in a culture obsessed by material success and display. Hence, there is an absence of cultural interest in the "lifestyles of the destitute and forlorn" that often crosses the threshold from indifference to disdain—even disgust—all of which are reminiscent of the comments made by Hawthorne about John Treeo.

The lifestyles of the affluent are widely embraced, thereby establishing an "enviable visibility" to their wealth, cars, homes, and pampered existences. To the contrary, the difficulties of a life lived in poverty with all its associated hardships are vanquished to invisibility for most Americans, yet these demands are ever present for the poor. The burden they impose is a seminal force that frames the social experience of their lives. This struggle not only defines the ways of life in poverty but, for patients and families, explicitly shapes the patterns by which they face the end of life.

I have stressed that financial success is a standard by which personal status is measured. Similarly, financial want is a wellspring of social stigma and personal shame. For the most part, and most interestingly, the dying poor I came to know complained little about economic inequality. More often than not, they accepted their economic situation without lament. Given the broader social context of rejection and stigma, it seemed especially striking that they expressed little hostility about the stigma of poverty. They were never embarrassed by their living conditions, nor did they take offense at the fact that I enjoyed far greater material privileges than they could imagine. When they did express discontent and frustration, it was always within the context of real financial hardship, worry, and deprivation. Typically, when this occurred, government bureaucracies and their associated hassles were involved.

Their economic concerns were many, ranging from being unable to pay bills to anxiety about the inability of their loved ones to "make it" after they died. In a relentless way, just as there was no reprieve from terminal illness, there was no escape from the consequences of being poor:

> **The financial worry overflows into other stuff that I have got to do. I say I've got to do, but I don't guess I've got to do any of it. But that financial situation controls my other parts of my life. The financial part of my life is in turmoil right now. I don't like that.**

For many the financial struggle was intense and persistent, as the following comments reveal.

> **I really don't have enough. Don't have enough to make ends meet. When I worked I had more money than I am getting now. SSI cut me down $28, that won't be nothing. Yeah, we are going to appeal it. Cause that ain't gonna work. You can't live off that.**

> **I don't have a lot of money, because if I did I'd have my bill paid at County.**

> **I really don't have enough.**

> **I don't have enough to make ends meet.**

> **I don't have enough. I don't have a job.**

Fear, anxiety, worry, and, perhaps, a feeling of icy terror stabbing at the heart are common parts of the experience of dying, regardless of economic or social status. For the dying poor, however, suffering at the end of life can be worsened. The grip of poverty often increases the difficulty and harshness of dying. It adds not only an additional layer of stress but also precipitates its own unique indignities.

The point is that poverty imposes harm to both patients and loved ones. Let us return briefly to the story of Mr. White, who, you will remember, was dying from esophageal cancer. Although he worked conscientiously all his life, the job he had had for the last twenty-nine years did not provide health benefits or a pension. His financial struggles were real and played an important part in defining not only his life and death but also in his wife's ability to grieve his death with dignity. Mr. White died in the county nursing home on a Friday morning. Despite not having the money to bury him, Mrs. White had the body removed to a neighborhood funeral home. There, the body remained for five days while the family scrambled to find a way to afford the cost of the funeral. Meanwhile, Mrs. White's grief over the death of her husband was intensified by feelings of shame and bewilderment. Finally, on the following Tuesday, an arrangement was made with the trustee's office that provided a "pauper's funeral service." This situation is not atypical in the world of the inner-city poor. Burial expenses are a great concern for many:

Our biggest worry is paying off the cemetery.

Another dying person, whose eyes were clouded in tears, not because he was dying but because he was worried about funeral expenses, drove the point home:

> My one worry or concern? The expenses. . . . I can't get insurance. I thought I'd go down there and pay so much to set up my own funeral, pay them $5 a month.

In the world of the more affluent, the idea of paying $5 a month to preplan a funeral would be ludicrous. In this man's world, however, it was all he could envision and afford. He frowned and continued:

> It shouldn't be so hard on her to try to get it paid. I am sad because we can't get no insurance.

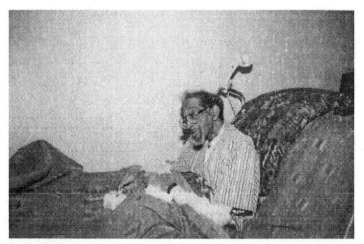

Reverend Brian laments the indifference of the rich in America to the hardships of the poor.

Funerals are important in the world of the dying poor. I have attended viewings and funeral services for many patients and have found them to be full of energy and communal presence. In the African-American community, especially, funerals are celebratory events steeped in ritual, with those in attendance dressed stylishly and elegantly. Most of the funeral homes in the inner city are lavishly appointed and provide a stark contrast to the neighborhoods in which they are located. A plush setting in which to say good-bye is important. As many expressed, they wanted to be buried with class and dignity. Ask dying poor persons about their wishes for their funerals and they will typically respond, "I just want to be put away well." Probe as to why, and they will likely answer, "So I don't bring shame and humiliation on my family." This fear of humiliation is related to the very real concern that they cannot afford a "proper funeral." There can be no doubt that financial strain affects the lives of patients and their loved ones, and worrying about money intensifies their emotional stress.

> **Just really the funeral burden is the worst for me.**
>
> **It's more of a pressure when you have someone sick with people harassing you about money. It becomes the biggest straining of all. . . . That's more of a stress than his sickness.**

Poverty also affects, on a regular basis, the daily experience of being seriously ill and imposes special demands on the lives of patients and families. Although a major purpose of the public hospital is to provide health care for the under- and uninsured, the rigmarole of bureaucracy must still be dealt with. Despite the gratitude of many for the care received, bureaucratic regulations add to a sense of frustration and disempowerment. One patient, who had been refused an appointment to an oncology clinic because he did not have $25 for copayment, was sent to the financial services office for processing into the "indigent program." He wandered around the hospital, somewhat lost and feeling dizzy and wobbly. As it turns out, his blood sugar was severely elevated at the time which contributed to his disorientation. Fortunately, while wandering the hallways he was approached by a volunteer, who was able to accompany him to the financial office, assist in getting him enrolled in the program, and then escort him back to the clinic, where he was seen later that day. The patient downplayed the situation and said, "It's always like that out here." Others feel more anger about the difficulty of navigating their way through the maze of bureaucracy at County:

> **He's home dying while I am running around with all you here [County], come get this paper . . . prove this . . . prove that.**
>
> **Well, I am 100% indigent . . . look at those bottles over, there is probably one-third of them that I have to buy at the pharmacy because County doesn't have them.**

A lot goes on in the world of the dying poor. Not only does financial deprivation remove their experiences from the emotional and social interest of more affluent Americans, the ugliness of dying in a culture of denial deepens their "invisibility." Ironically, however, despite enormous social estrangement from mainstream American life, the dying poor face many of the same worries that more affluent families confront. These similarities have to do with a certain universality of human experience that transcends class, status, and culture at the end of life. Among the common experiences of the poor and the nonpoor are the profound emotional effects of the body being destroyed by disease, pervasive anxiety, concern about loved ones, and the intense need to retain a sense of hope.

The poor, like most dying persons, were often horrified at the physical effects of disease. It was difficult for them to become "witnesses and spectators" to their own bodily devolution. In a most human way, it was difficult for these patients to suffer the indignities of physical deterioration. As their bodies started to fail, they worried about how they looked or appeared to others:

> My hair started coming out in clumps when I was in the shower and I just started shrieking.

> I don't want to be all crumpled up; a haggy-looking old thing dying. I want to go with a little peace and dignity.

> I don't like to go out anywhere. . . . I'm worried about how I look.

> My biggest concern as far as this here death thing is again like I said what I went through with my brother. He had lung cancer and he died from lung cancer and he was taking chemo just like me. This has happened a little over two years ago and I can remember him lying in the bed and I would think to myself—wow, he went from a robust active man to a man who looked like he just got out of a concentration camp. That's what I don't want to happen to me.

> I have lost about forty pounds since the time I was diagnosed with it. People look at you.

Despite the fact that the dying poor are socially distant from the mainstream culture, the worries they have when their bodies are dismantled by disease and dying are not always unique to their world. Their anxiety over loss of physical integrity is natural, perhaps universal. Certainly, it is also consistent with the values that shape more affluent Americans. It is no secret in our culture of materialism that attractive physical appearance matters, and it matters in ways that extend beyond mere physical meaning. Beauty, in the American cultural worldview, is associated with success, self-confidence, personal competence, and even likeability. In this context, physical beauty enhances social status, whereas ugliness diminishes it. My interest in raising this issue is not to offer a critique of the overimportance of physical appearance in American life. Rather, it is to emphasize that the dying poor feel deeply the cultural and social stigma of bodily deterioration. In this regard, the worries expressed by patients show a paradox wherein the poor, who are in many ways disassociated from the broader culture, are still influenced by and connected to it.

The deterioration of the body while anticipating death also has a profound emotional impact on both individuals and families. For many patients, the greatest challenge is to find meaning and emotional comfort while living with the fear of physical deterioration and death. It was difficult for many patients to accept the fact they could no longer do the things they used to do. Mr. McMann, for example, longed to go fishing just one more time. Unfortunately, the rapid spread of his disease and relentless pain prevented him from being able to go on that last fishing trip. He regretted this fact often during the last months of his life, all of which were spent in a nursing home. As we will see in greater detail in subsequent chapters, living in the shadow of death was an ever-present source of distress, yet many endured dying's tribulations privately and, for the most part, without raising a fuss. In private conversations they would, however, often freely express their concerns, appearing grateful for the opportunity to voice what they were feeling and had largely internalized. Their words are simply and painfully to the point:

> I get depressed. . . . Lord knows that I am not ready yet.
>
> See, I never had the chicken pox, measles, mumps, or nothing like that. Then, the first time you get sick and are told you have cancer—I was devastated.
>
> I was sick and stressed out. I had a breakdown. It's hard. Hard.
>
> I just don't talk much about it at all, that makes it better.
>
> I'm not going to talk to you about my cancer, honey.
>
> Well, I think I went into a bit of depression because I started feeling sorry for myself.
>
> I just don't think about it.

These sentiments of loss and emotional devastation are normal in most dying persons, regardless of income or social status. The chaos and financial want of living in poverty, however, add an additional burden that can deepen emotional loss and suffering.

Nevertheless, although poverty shapes the process of dying in ways that can make the experience more stressful, its impact is not always negative. In this regard, another paradox becomes evident: the enormous difficulties of dying, intensified by the legacy of living in poverty, are sometimes eased by the character-deepening experiences of a life lived in poverty. Even though dying precipitated deep emotional worry for some, others displayed a remarkable peacefulness in dying. Indeed, an impressive number of the dying poor faced their deaths with acceptance and equanimity:

> No, I am not afraid. None of us were put on this earth to live forever.

One doctor told me that I would live two years. One doctor asked me how did I feel about it? Well, I look at it this way: everybody's got to die sometime.

Everybody in every walk of life has got to go through it.

I am not mad at anyone for what I have. I know that I have it. I don't have a problem with it.

Some people say why did it have to happen to me—why me? I don't feel that way.

Something seemingly contradictory happens in the world of the dying poor. Despite extensive financial and social disempowerment, many possess a spirit and strength that enable them to confront their suffering and dying with remarkable composure. I was often struck by how deep this hidden power ran in their lives. Honestly, there were times when I—from the vantage point of my personal and professional privileges—was bewildered at how easily some patients gave themselves over to the process of dying. Sometimes I would even joke with colleagues about how I wanted to "shake them, let them know that they are dying and that they ought to be afraid." I often remarked about how difficult it would be for us to be in their place. "Unimaginable," we would say, knowing full well that we would likely suffer great emotional and personal distress were we to hear the bad news of a terminal diagnosis. Here, again, we come to another irony. As highly educated professionals, we were confident in our abilities to self-advocate. We were also in a privileged financial position compared to these patients, yet, for all our personal, professional, and financial empowerment, in some ways we felt we lacked the resources to cope with the end of life with the same confidence and calmness that many patients displayed. This paradox, while perplexing, is simply put: the disempowered are often more empowered in facing the burden of suffering, disease, and death than are those more empowered and advantaged. Perhaps, in this regard, the sense of control—of choice—that more affluent individuals possess is, in some ways, an illusion that is revealed throughout the dying process.

I puzzled extensively over this unexpected, eye-opening discovery. In fact, the poise that some patients displayed was not only remarkable but also taught much about their lives. The lessons to be learned seemed clear. Although the terrible burdens of poverty made life difficult for these patients, these same burdens cultivated a certain toughness of personality that served them well during the trials of dying. When one is living at the financial edge, where daily life is shaped by constant financial struggle, "a cancer diagnosis is just one more bad thing to happen this week." In a sense, the sting of serious disease is "softened" by the fact that the poor already are facing so many hardships. Contrariwise, in a life of privilege and advantage, dying threatens deeply because there is so much more to lose. In addition, when one lives and succeeds in an affluent and empowered life, perhaps one is likely to resist surrendering to "God's will" all the more tenaciously. In that framework, in which one is self-assertive, optimistic about the future, and largely in control of one's life, it is all the more difficult to make the emotional adjustment that is necessary for acceptance of life's end. On the other hand, the dying poor have lived most of their lives in surrender—particularly a forced surrender to the hardships of poverty. Although poverty in inner-city America resembles little the experience of being poor in sub-Saharan Africa, for example, it nonetheless inflicts deep and consistent harm to the lives it touches. Thus, the sufferings of poverty, although punitive and violent in attacking human dignity, ironically can cultivate a certain strength of character and depth of personality that are particularly valuable in helping some develop a sense of calm and serenity in dying.

I am not suggesting these patients wanted to die. Hope, as it is in all human experience, was central to their lives and gave them reassurance. They hoped for a lot of things, including being able to defeat their diseases. For some hope was kindled by belief in "technological miracles," as they placed great faith in the curative powers of medicine. Especially prominent in this group were African Americans. I regularly witnessed both patients and families demanding that everything possible be done. Attached to this attitude was a reluctance to accept the medical judgment of physicians that the best decision was to withdraw treatment or not to extend it. Some, especially if a fatal prognosis was given, were even reluctant to accept the medical diagnosis. One family, for example, was quite mistrusting of the intensive care unit physicians who had determined that the eighty-year-old matriarch of the family was brain dead. They bitterly fought the doctors and refused to give permission to have her withdrawn from the ventilator for eight days. These were days filled with anger and unsatisfactory dialogue between the family and the physicians. After permission was finally granted and life support was withdrawn, it seemed as if all the involved parties went away frustrated and unhappy.

It is not unusual when these situations arise for staff to struggle to understand why patients or families find it difficult to accept a diagnosis and prognosis. Staff are also often perplexed at the mistrust and intense emotional reactions displayed by many families. One nurse told about another patient who was "literally brain dead," but once again the family "refused to believe it. They would bring tapes in," she said, "and wail and scream. That part was real difficult to understand and deal with." What is being reflected here is a deep cultural divide between the personal and cultural background of patients and families and the professional worldview of care providers. The result is a difficult tension between the insistent technological hopefulness of a disempowered population and how their "unreasonableness" flies in the face of the medical facts as understood by physicians and nurses.

This mindset of patients and families is also partially related to a natural inclination, in this day and age, to fight death as resolutely as possible. The following sentiments expressed by many of the dying poor are part of a psychological and emotional response that is not tied exclusively to class or race. Instead, these words reflect an unrealistic optimism that has much more to do with human personality, especially in an age of death denial:

> I'm gonna beat it.

> I try to keep a positive attitude that I am gonna recover from this. . . . Right now I don't find anything scary about it. Because I truly believe that I am gonna recover.

> I still have this feeling of immortality sometimes. . . . I still have this feeling like, oh well, yeah I've got lung cancer and they told me I am going to die—but oh yeah, oh well, maybe not.

> Now, right now I think I am going to beat it. Some days I feel that it's running, but for the most part, I am still positive that I am going to win.

> As long as we don't dwell over the sickness, you can overcome it.

> I think that my future is going to be wonderful. I really do. I think it is going to be wonderful.

These attitudes, typical throughout our culture, invoke components of denial, optimism, and selective understanding. They involve crafting a positive, life-affirming view toward the future that involves evasion and avoidance of truth. This attitude was more or less apparent in some patients and families, depending on pre-existing personal and psychological dynamics, and was not necessarily influenced by the social variables of race, class, or status. In addition, this type of optimistic, hopeful attitude was also changeable in patients and families. It would often be experienced alongside despair and depression, creating a very fluid dynamic wherein patients would oscillate between feelings of optimism and pessimism, week by week, day by day, hour by hour.

As already indicated, some attitudes and expressions of hope were uniquely connected to the inner-city African-American experience. In this particular frame of mind, technological dependence was galvanized with both religious faith and the cultural background of the African-American community. The result was a strong sentiment that demanded "everything" be done to attack the disease, even after clinical judgment had determined that curative intervention would be useless.

There are three driving forces behind this attitude. The first has to do with mistrust. For understandable reasons, the African-American patient population is often suspicious of the intentions and motives of their physicians, who are often white and far removed from their own cultural experiences. In some ways, because the end of life creates so much stress, this mistrust and disconnection is intensified throughout the experience of dying.

Second, these individuals have felt the sting of poverty throughout much of their lives. As part of this experience, they have lived with rejection and endured the many frustrations of dealing with "welfare bureaucracies." As part of their way of coping with dying, having lived a life of financial and cultural disempowerment, they aggressively seek to access and receive every possible service they can. In this framework, medical advice to not begin new treatments or to discontinue current ones may be interpreted as one more form of deprivation.

The third underlying factor involves the place and power of religion in their lives. For many, faith in God is the foundation of life. It provides the strength that enables them to survive poverty. In this faith, they believe not only in the goodness of God but also in His mightiness. These truly are individuals who believe in the possibilities of miracles and in God's power to cure. Their demand for aggressive, life-prolonging technological interventions comes directly from faith. As a result, some patients and families wanted their physicians to prolong life as long as possible. In doing so, by using their God-given skills, they would provide the time necessary for God to work a miracle. In this way the certainty of belief in God's power defined what they thought the job of physicians should be. As suggested earlier, when patients, families, and pastors insisted on treatment in medically futile situations, they were often seen as intransigent by the medical staff. This conflict between professional medical opinion and the faith of this population often led to misunderstandings and difficult interactions among patients, families, pastors, and physicians. Physicians from very different personal and professional circumstances, often saw this viewpoint as clinically "ridiculous." Thus, the differing perspectives between physicians and patients, coupled with an absence of empathy and poor communication skills on the part of some doctors, only served to inflame already existing feelings of mistrust. In these situations, as suggested earlier, it often seemed that all parties went away dissatisfied.

However, not all African-American patients demanded technologically zealous interventions. In fact, a good many were suspicious of life-prolonging treatment and worried about its associated indignities. In this framework patients who had heard or experienced the horrors of modern dying were frightened and anxious about technologically driven abuses of dignity. The words of several patients express this fear directly:

> I just don't want to be on that machine.

> I am not going to have my family, my children, my wife, anybody coming up there and seeing me hooked up to no machine.

> I am not going to let them put something down my throat, push on my chest. Nothing is going to bring me back because you have to go home to Him.

> I'm not going to get on no machine. That's it!

For these patients and others like them, hope assumed a different meaning. It was not connected to the miraculous, life-saving capabilities of technology or even spiritual salvation. For them, hope had to do with quality of life. They hoped for a "no-pain death" with "none of that suffering crap." They hoped their loved ones would be "provided for after I die." They hoped that the presence of caring others would see them into their deaths: "My family is very important to me. They are all I have got. They are here when I need them. My wife never leaves my side no matter what." The priority for these individuals was related to living as well as possible, given their acceptance that they were going to die.

Thus, whether it was to "go back south one more time and see my family," "go fishing," or "see my grandchildren graduate," the hopeful focus revolved around relief of suffering, spiritual reconciliation, family relationships, reducing financial distress, and being able to look forward to enjoyable things as much as possible. All of this was part of an effort to stem the tide of loss and find reassurance that life still had purpose. As one person perceptively expressed, hopeful optimism is not always related to treatment, remission, and cure, but cherishing life:

> **There is a life beyond medical problems. Whenever you talk to them about something that makes them happy—flowers, blue skies, blue waters, kids, anything—that's the most wonderful thing in the world.**

In summary, the world of the dying poor is filled with strain, tension, and contradictory expressions that often play against one another. Some of these tensions and contradictions typically unfold throughout all human experience; others are uniquely the product of inner-city poverty in shaping the experience of dying. Most important of all is that the sufferings and joys of poor people seem to matter little in a culture driven by icons of material success, making it all the more urgent to tell these stories. Listening to their stories is a way of respecting and honoring their lives. It also offers a reminder that the poor, although inhabitants of an alien place in a culture of materialism, share a sense of humanity and spirit that connects them to even the most affluent among us. Finally, it reveals a collective spirit that remains unspoken and unheard, the whispers of which portray the richness and dignity of their lives.

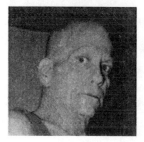

DYING IN THE PUBLIC HOSPITAL SYSTEM: INSTITUTIONAL ARRANGEMENTS AND PROVIDER PERSPECTIVES

Although there is much that is complex about dying poor, choosing which hospital system will direct medical care is simple: there is only one hospital in Indianapolis that provides comprehensive care for the poor.

The Institutional Landscape

Originally constructed as a military hospital during the Civil War, what now is called County Health Services (CHS) has been through many changes in its 140-year history. As City Hospital it began its mission to serve the poor in 1866 and has continued to the present day.

CHS is now part of a large university medical center that includes a university hospital, Veteran's Administration hospital, and children's hospital, along with medical, nursing, and allied health sciences schools, medical research facilities, and a library. The County Hospital complex takes up several city blocks, and the medical center covers nearly one square mile. Like many other hospital systems, the university and children's hospitals have recently merged with another hospital. These two hospital campuses, about 1.5 miles apart from each other, are connected by a multimillion-dollar monorail transportation system that runs through the surrounding poor urban areas and allow health-care providers to commute easily between the two centers. County Hospital, while physically located on the medical center campus and staffed by university physicians, was not part of the merger.

The mission of County in serving patients differs from that of private hospitals, and last year County operated at a $20 million deficit.

The buildings that constitute this public hospital system are similar to those in most medical centers. Some of the buildings are more than 140 years old, with original floors and banisters, but are continuously remodeled and enlarged to meet the needs of modern medicine. Hallways are long and curve strangely; it is easy to get lost. It is not uncommon to see patients being transported from one place to another in handcuffs accompanied by prison guards, readily identifiable by their bright yellow or orange uniforms. Signs in the hospital direct you to the burn unit, intensive care, ER, ambulatory surgery, detention, and the mental health center. Other buildings, such as the primary care center, birthing center, burn unit, and nursing home, are as new and modern as are any in the country.

The patient population at CHS is predominantly poor, undereducated, and racially diverse. Only six percent of the hospital's patients have commercial insurance, so the hospital is filled with the city's sick and indigent. Although all hospitals in this system care for some indigent patients, the public hospital receives more than seventy-five percent of its revenues from Medicaid and Medicare payments. It draws its patients from urban areas that contain and encircle all these hospitals in the center of the city as well as those living in the county's eastern and western working-class neighborhoods.

Thanks to all the ethicists, researchers, and scholars at the medical center as well as the physicians, nurses, and other health-care providers who work there, CHS is a vibrant, intellectually stimulating environment. It is also a prime teaching site for the school of medicine, as it provides a pool of patients with whom students, interns, and residents advance their knowledge and skills. For dying individuals, however, CHS is obviously something quite different. To them it is the place where they or their loved ones were diagnosed with a fatal illness, where they receive treatment, and sometimes the place of their death. It is a place that often infuriates and alienates, but it is also the place upon which they are dependent. Sometimes, as noted in the previous chapter, it is a place for which they are deeply grateful. Regardless of the type of experiences individuals and families have in this system, County plays a significant part in their lives and deaths. This chapter describes the public hospital system, how it functions for dying patients, and health-care providers' views of their attempts to serve the poor through the dying process. It provides a picture of what any patient entering the system can typically expect to find.

Although patients and their families often live fairly close to the hospital, getting there can be decidedly difficult for them. To begin with, many patients do not have reliable cars or are too sick to drive. They may arrange rides from friends or family, but many of them also do not have reliable transportation or dependable childcare to make it possible for them to perform such a favor. Patients can take a city bus to the hospital, but that means they must be physically able to leave their house and get to the bus stop. Their ride may be very long and typically will require changing buses. Some charitable organizations arrange to drive patients to their physician visits, but this service is limited in the ways it can help patients. For instance, the Little Red Door is an agency that provides transportation to the hospital, but this must be arranged in advance, making it unhelpful for acute exacerbations of an illness that require immediate medical attention. In addition, this kind of transportation is provided only from the curb to the hospital entrance, which leaves the most difficult aspects of getting out of the house and from the door of the hospital to the appropriate clinic to the often-debilitated patient.

When it is impossible for patients to get themselves to the hospital or arrange a ride, they are left with two options. First, they may choose not go to the hospital or clinic, leaving them without needed medical care. And, frankly, to the frustration and chagrin of their doctors, some do choose not to keep regularly scheduled appointments. Second, they may call an ambulance and be transported to the emergency department. In this case they will receive medical care, but not by their primary physicians and at a huge cost.

Once delivered to the door of the hospital, the seriously ill patient still has the challenge of getting to different areas of the hospital required for monthly blood draws, X-rays, clinic visits, and pharmacy needs. Jodi, the palliative care nurse at County, described one of her patients who parked in the parking garage and then walked a great distance to the pain clinic on the far side of the hospital. The woman knew she was dying and wanted no extraordinary measures taken to save her life. As she walked to her clinic, she got very tired and short of breath. Her greatest fear was that she would collapse in the hospital and that medical personnel would resuscitate her, so she clutched her advance directive in her hand as she walked. (Like most indigent patients, this woman never complained about her trouble with the long walk, which was discovered purely by chance. When it was discovered, she was told that it was permissible for her to park in a special parking lot right next to the pain clinic, which she did. Before the chance encounter that brought the situation to light, she was completely unaware that this option was available to her).

I also remember waiting for Lucille Angel one morning in the oncology clinic, wondering why she was more than an hour late for her scheduled appointment. Finally, she emerged from the elevator alone. The sight of her was striking. Her wig covered her hairless head, and she looked ashen and on the verge of collapse while she moved her walker forward four inches at a time. It cannot be emphasized strongly enough that getting to the clinic or doctor's office for medical care is an especially difficult challenge for many indigent patients. For these who are seriously ill and dying, the obstacles are even more formidable.

Dying patients have contact with several parts of CHS. Arguably, the most important of these is the emergency room, which often is the front gate to health care for the poor. The primary care and specialty clinics in which patients are diagnosed and treated as their diseases progress are also important parts of the system of care, as are the community health centers that provide primary care services in inner-city neighborhoods. When they have acute exacerbations of their diseases, they may also be admitted to the medical or intensive care areas of the hospital. In their experience in CHS, poor patients encounter a vast array of health-care providers and students. In fact, the students, interns, residents, and specialty doctors change so often in this system of care that it is unusual for patients and families to remember the names of doctors who took care of them.

The organization of medical students and physicians and the roles they play in caring for patients in an academic medical center are complex and can be quite confusing. The senior physicians in this system of care are called staff physicians. They are permanently on staff and hold titles of assistant, associate, or full professors in the university. The staff rotate through different "services" on a monthly basis. A particular specialty is in charge of different services. Physicians see patients both in the hospital in sections referred to as wards and in out-patient settings called clinics. Staff rotate throughout different hospitals many times and are in charge of the Service to which they are assigned, which means they are ultimately responsible for all patient care. They may treat patients on their own, conduct rounds during which the medical team discusses the management of each patient each day, and also "staff" patients. "Staffing" means they listen to the assessment of the patient and the plan for treatment generated by fellows, residents, and third and fourth year medical students, who in reality provide most of the one-on-one care for patients at County.

Fellows are at the next-lower level in this hierarchy. They have completed a three to seven year residency and are receiving further specialty training. For example, if they were trained in internal medicine, they might go on for two or three more years of training in oncology, cardiology, pulmonology, or other specialties. Fellows see patients only in their area of specialty and spend longer blocks of time in particular clinics.

Residents are at the next level of training and authority. Residents have completed medical school and so are officially medical doctors. Most residencies last three years, but some may last as long as seven. It is usually at the end of the first year that residents obtain a license to practice medicine independently and are not required by law to pursue further training. In contrast to the fellows, who spend as many as six months at a time on one particular service, residents are required to rotate through their own specialty and other related fields on a monthly basis. Fifty percent or more of an internal medicine resident's rotations will be "wards," that is, managing patients in the hospital on the medicine service. The rest of their time will be spent rotating through the subspecialties of internal medicine (pulmonology, infectious disease, cardiology, oncology, renal, etc.), primarily seeing these patients in the hospital and, less commonly, in out-patient clinics. Residents, therefore, have patients for one month at a time and turn over their patients to the incoming resident at the end of each rotation. As I will indicate, this creates a situation wherein lack of continuity in care becomes a problem. In short, residents provide most of the hands-on care in an academic hospital, examining patients, performing procedures, and ordering medicines and tests. Their work is supervised by their assigned staff daily.

At the bottom of the medical hierarchy are the third and fourth year medical students. Medical students rotate through various services and hospitals for two years, working most closely with the residents. They observe and participate in rounds and write daily notes on the patients assigned to their service. Although they have already completed two years of medical school, these rotations are typically their first experiences in taking care of patients.

Many residents are also assigned to a clinic for at least half a day per week. A clinic is an out-patient setting in which patients are followed for chronic conditions. At the school of medicine, medicine residents are assigned a group of clinic patients as interns and are expected to follow those patients throughout the three-year residency. This is intended to foster continuity of care, although, in reality, patients may see a different doctor every time they come to the clinic. When the patient's primary physician leaves at the end of three years, the patient is assigned to an incoming intern. Thus, continuity can be disrupted at any point in an illness. Some patients are assigned primarily to the more experienced staff physicians instead of an intern and have greater chances of seeing a single physician throughout the dying process.

Many of the patients I met throughout this project were initially assigned to an internal medicine intern in this out-patient clinic. Many of the patients were also seen in specialty clinics, most notably the oncology clinic. In the oncology clinic, there is one physician on staff who sees patients each week. Two nurses work there permanently and provide the most consistency. In addition, other staff physicians rotate through the clinic periodically. Oncology fellows come through for six months at a time, and internal medicine residents rotate through for one-month intervals. This changing coterie of physicians means that patients do not always see the same people when they come to the clinic. Thus, attempts to build intimate relationships are often foiled, and, frankly, as already noted, many patients do not even know the names of their doctors in specialty clinics.

Clinics are supposed to run for four hours. They are always full, and then additional patients who need to be seen are "worked in," which slows the rate at which patients are seen. Both medicine and oncology clinics are generally very busy and often run two or more hours behind. It often takes patients between four and five hours to complete a clinic visit. It also means that physicians who are scheduled to work from 8:00 AM to noon are working in the clinic from 8:00 AM to 1:30 PM or 2:00 PM. During acute exacerbations of their illnesses, patients often visit the emergency department, where they will be treated by still a different physician, medical student, or resident. As already noted, many indigent people use the emergency room (ER) as their primary doctor's office. It is the first place they think of when not feeling well. It is not unusual for patients to wait seven to eight hours to see a doctor in the ER if the situation is not deemed an emergency.

In fact, most visits to the ER involve situations that are less than life threatening. This is nowhere more the case than in the world of the inner-city poor. The ER is, in reality, the "doctor's office" for many. Consider John Evans, an alcoholic who hustled and lived in the streets. Diagnosed with liver cancer, he became a patient of legendary status among the ER doctors, using the ER eighty-nine times over a ninety-day period. He would often come in the morning, be discharged, go get drunk, and return later in the day dazed by alcohol, having forgotten he had already been there earlier. Unlike Norm on *Cheers* who was not just a regular presence on his bar stool but one who was beloved, John was familiar but oftentimes despised. Many of the staff in the chaotic world of the public hospital's ER, in frustration and work-related stress, have been known to degrade the personhood of the indigent patients who frequent the ER. It is not unusual for comments such as "What does this asshole want now," or "I can't believe that this scumbag is back," or "When are you queers ever going to learn" (said to a patient with AIDS), to be made by ER staff about the "John Evanses of the world."

However, as disturbing as is this portrait of care, there is another side to the care delivered in the county hospital and ER that is as virtuous as the above is regrettable. There are physicians, nurses, social workers, and chaplains who would not work anywhere else. For example, there is a staff physician in the ER who recently left a lucrative practice in a private hospital in Arizona to come to inner-city Indianapolis for the express purpose of caring for the poor. Ask him about his approach to coping with the frustration and chaos of the public hospital ER, and he will talk about his theory of "compassion epidemiology," whereby he compares the personal strain imposed on him by the most difficult of patients, those like John Evans, to the suffering those individuals endure daily in their poverty-ridden lives. "There's no comparison," he states. "No matter how irritated I get, no matter how tired I am, all I have to do is to remind myself of the struggles this population face in their lives outside the hospital, and everything comes back into perspective. It is the formula by which I continually rekindle empathy for these patients." This physician regularly uses this strategy to teach the value and practice of empathy to residents and students, "with mixed success," he comments. As you can imagine, the patients who are Dr. L's "regulars" in the ER absolutely love him because of the respect he shows them.

Another example of virtuous care of the dying poor involved a patient and doctor who met in the ER. In fact, this sets the gold standard for the virtuous practice of medicine. Tina was a young woman in her mid-thirties whose body was being devastated beyond description by malignant melanoma. She was in exquisite pain when she came to the ER. She was terrified and emotionally alarmed, not just of dying but of being alone. Tina had no family in her life. She had been on her own, surviving the streets as best she could, since she was thirteen. Having lived deprived of stable, loving relationships throughout her life, she worried that she would die abandoned and neglected. The physician who saw her in the emergency room made her two promises: if it were possible, her pain would be controlled, and she would not come to the end of her life isolated and alone. Both promises were kept. Her pain was eased by morphine. Her associated hallucinations, most notably of frogs that were terrifyingly real to her, were eased by the regular caring presence of the nurse at her bedside in the hospital, who worked in close connection with the physician. The second promise was perhaps a bit more complicated to keep. How does one ensure that a person, who for all practical purposes is alone in the world, will not die alone? The answer provided by the doctor was quite extraordinary. She took the patient home and along with the help of her husband, also a physician in the public hospital, and the palliative care team nurse, she cared for Tina until her death a week later.

To complete the story of John Evans, "the grand old man of the ER," through extraordinary effort the palliative care social worker was able to convince a local street minister to provide housing for Mr. Evans in a local hotel. There, he was regularly fed, visited, and attended to. Ironically, because of the efforts of empathic individuals at the County Hospital, hospice, and the local community, this "asshole" lived the final four weeks of his life connected to caring others. In small but momentous ways the epitaph of John Treeo is, perhaps, being rewritten—not for all, but for some—by those caring professionals who work, by choice, in the public hospital.

Once seen in the ER, patients are then either released or admitted to the hospital. If a patient is admitted, he or she is then "managed" by a completely different group of physicians. The physicians at the clinics in which patients are seen will not know what happened in the hospital until they review the patient's chart before their next clinic visit or unless they are contacted directly by the ER physicians.

Patients themselves have different assessments of the hospital system as a whole. According to patient satisfaction surveys, they are overwhelmingly positive about their experiences at CHS. Some of the dying patients see visits to the hospital or clinic as a time to socialize and, perhaps, to show to the outside world that they are still holding their lives together. For example, Reverend Brian would wear a three-piece suit when visiting the oncology clinic. Mrs. Angel was always nicely dressed and groomed at the hospital. Often, patients' attempts to look nice are greeted enthusiastically by the nursing and secretarial staff, who comment on their styled hair and attractive outfits. The nursing staff, despite a frenetic pace and work environment, also attempt to make patients comfortable during chemotherapy, which is administered in a private room in the clinic. One of the clinic nurses, for example, always made sure Mrs. Angel had a VCR and John Wayne movies to watch while she received chemotherapy, for which she and her family were always appreciative.

Although many patients derive some pleasure from their visits to the hospital, the fact of the matter is that dying in such a complex bureaucracy can be particularly frightening. It requires patience during waits in the ER, waiting in the pharmacy for medications, navigating the immense physical layout of the hospital (patients regularly wander the hallways lost, trying to find their place of appointment), along with trying to remember the many physicians, nurses, and social workers who will become part of their lives. Most patients are rarely able to distinguish among students, interns, residents, or staff physicians. Although close personal doctor–patient relationships are the ideal, fragmented care that lacks continuity is the unfortunate norm.

Reverend Brian and his wife are a good example of a couple who successfully learned to navigate the system to best serve their needs. They had recently had several deaths in their family that had taken place at County. They therefore felt they had experience with the hospital and the way it worked. They made lists of questions before they came to an appointment. They were very clear about what they wanted to know and how they would make decisions regarding that knowledge. For important matters, such as whether to have a "do not resuscitate" order on the chart, the Brians refused to talk to anyone but their primary care physician, with whom they had developed a relationship and who they absolutely loved and trusted.

Many others, however, never find such effective means of controlling the chaotic environment. Although a few may lash out at caregivers in frustration, most bottle up their feelings and never ask for help. Still others drop out of the system, foregoing necessary medical care.

A Provider Profile

A tremendous variety of people work at CHS. Some are required to work there as part of their training. Those required to rotate through County during medical school or residency do not necessarily have a commitment to serve the health-care needs of the poor. In fact, they may resent giving costly medical care to indigent patients. As one staff physician noted, "Unfortunately, in our profession there are a lot of judgmental people, very judgmental, who, as soon as they leave the room and as soon as they leave the family, will make a statement like, 'That piece of trash is better off dead.'" As already stated, indigent patients throughout the system are sometimes referred to as "scumbags" or "dirtballs" and talked about in disparaging language.

In sharp contrast to these negative attitudes are the feelings of the staff physicians, nurses, and social workers who choose to work with the poor. Some choose to work at County out of a sense of service and mission. Others find the environment stimulating and note that there is something intrinsically interesting and rewarding about working with an urban, indigent population.

One of the most unanticipated things I found at County was that many of the permanent staff are drawn to the patient population. An internist described the feelings she has for her patients as a group. "I care for the most interesting, wonderful group of patients. I have a woman who is an executive for American Express. (Remember that six percent of patients have commercial insurance.) [Another] patient just died of carcinoma in the hospital. He was an I.V. drug user, lots of felony charges, and he was still married to the woman he has been married to for thirty-eight years, and I really respected him as a person." She is continuously "humbled by people with modest means doing what I thought was a Herculean effort," and she thinks this makes her a better daughter, a better parent, and a better doctor. Recently she told the story of an African-American family who took care of their grandmother who was stricken with Alzheimer's. "For three years they cared for her at home. It was just remarkable. I have a loving family that is educated and affluent, but I can't imagine them doing that for me. The strength of this family, and their faith, is a model for all of us."

Another provider said, "I tend to be more emotionally involved with the poorer population than I would with somebody who has money. Maybe I feel like that person never got a fair chance at life. Maybe that sounds silly or petty, but . . . I feel like they never got a true chance at life, or they never got a chance to have the nice things. Not just material things, but I just feel like they never got a chance to get the education or get the life experiences that go along with being able to have money." Another provider said, "I just generally prefer poor people. . . . I'm more comfortable at County than I am at University Hospital. I just always have drifted that way and feel connected that way." Yet another provider stated simply, "I'm here because I want to be here. I'm here because I consider it a privilege."

Providers who care for dying patients also consider that experience a kind of privilege that has both scientific and personal values. An oncologist involved in pharmaceutical research described these two reasons in a fairly typical way. "One is a scientific reason, because the bulk of my work is in a scientific laboratory trying to design the next generation of drugs that we might use. In addition, in order to make a new drug, the scientific hypothesis has to be relevant to an issue in clinical medicine. Therefore, to have knowledge of current clinical medicine I think is important for laboratory scientists. At the same time, I feel . . . humbled by patients who have cancer, and I have always considered it almost a privilege to listen to their story and to offer, if at all possible, some kind of relief for the last leg of a journey when a patient is actively dying. So, in an odd way, I find that personally rewarding."

The main difference providers note about indigent patients is that they communicate quite differently compared to patients who are more affluent. One physician reports, "When I go to University Hospital I have to deal with a lot more explanation to the family members, but for some reason when I am here, the family is not that aggressive in pursuing information. Patients and family members of the more educated patients will seek more and more information. While patients and family members of the more educated patients, and I have to say education is a key thing because I don't think it's money that is the issue . . . basically they don't ask many questions at all." As I will show in greater detail later, the disempowerment of the dying poor is a complicated matter that involves many factors. Of course, lack of education is relevant, but it misrepresents the nature and impact of poverty to suggest that lack of money is not related as well. Another provider said, "For the most part, families accept what we tell them. We don't lie to them and I think they accept it. A lot of times they don't ask a lot of questions probably because they don't know what kind of questions to ask. You tell them, 'This is what's going on. This is why it is going on. Do you have any questions?' 'No, I don't think so.' "

The lack of information gathering is in some ways appreciated by the staff because it makes giving bad or complicated information easier. "I mean, if the family of the patient is not interested in the rationale, then you don't have to explain the whole thing. That makes it easier for you, not to have to explain to the patient why you are dying, what the actual pathophysiology of your disease is, so you can understand. It is easier not to have to explain it . . . The educated patient not only questions but challenges your answers." Please keep these comments in mind as you read the patient narratives that will constitute the remaining chapters, for, indeed, they greatly challenge the assumption that indigent patients do not want detailed information. To the contrary, these narratives demonstrate that poor patients do want more information, and the quality of their lives is diminished because it often is not forthcoming.

In sum, these providers who choose to work in the public hospital are drawn to poor patients because they find them inherently interesting and because the experience of participating in care at the end of life is personally enriching and provides an opportunity to be of virtuous service to people who are especially vulnerable. Those with experience have a general idea of what should count as success, summed up by one experienced physician: "As long as I can feel that we did well, and if I feel that the medical system responded to them, and if I can have some sense that they died in the fashion that they chose, then I'm okay with that, even still being extremely distraught over certain deaths."

Noble professional motives, however, do not necessarily translate into effective communication and compassionate care from the patients' perspectives. What appear to be successful encounters to the health-care providers may not be judged as favorably by patients.

Many of the professional challenges in dealing with the dying poor do not stem from the fact that these physicians work in a county hospital system. Rather, they are the challenges specific to diagnosing and treating terminal conditions, which are common to all physicians who treat dying patients. Strangely enough, very few physicians receive useful medical training related to caring for dying patients, even in specialties such as oncology, which has a substantial segment of terminally ill patients. It is important to note, however, that lack of formal training is not equivalent to lack of socialization. There is a remarkable similarity in the practices that govern the ways physicians break bad news, communicate poor prognoses, and "manage" hope toward the end of life. These patterns are learned by watching others and by mild and informal professional censure when physicians stray very far away from the norm. These patterns may be referred to as a "culture of care" that gets passed on from older to younger physicians.

Most physicians share a vague ideal about the proper manner in which to disclose a terminal prognosis. They agree that a terminal prognosis is a serious matter and that it should not be "sprung" on the patient. Rather, physicians seek to break this kind of news gradually. Optimally, this is done in the context of a relationship that has evolved over time, but at County this may not be possible. Most physicians who suspect a terminal condition prefer not to talk about prognosis during their first visit with a patient. Unless the terminal disease process is in an acute stage and will rapidly lead to death, physicians prefer to have the opportunity to try to build a relationship before relating such bad news. At their first meeting with a patient, physicians do a physical exam and assess the patient's understanding of his or her disease and support system. However, they know that the real purpose of the first visit is to allow the patient to get used to them as their medical caregivers. An oncologist related, "My experience has been that people don't remember a lot of that first visit because they are still trying to get past me as a person they've never seen." Perhaps, on a deeper level, patients and families are trying to cope with the tidal wave of emotions that comes from a cancer diagnosis. Having the diagnosis delivered by a stranger seems to make the experience only more difficult to manage.

In addition, physicians believe they should provide their patients with complete disclosure of their medical condition in language the patient can understand. With the benefit of clearly conveyed information, they hope that the patient can make decisions best in accord with his or her values and goals. In considering patient stories in greater detail in subsequent chapters, it will be important to evaluate whether these ideals are actually achieved.

Many factors complicate or compromise the "ideal scenario." First and foremost, as we have already seen, it is often quite difficult to provide experienced care from a consistent caregiver in the public hospital system. Additionally, even with a consistent caregiver, the style and content of disclosure varies greatly from physician to physician. Full disclosure means vastly different things to different people, and often doctors seek refuge from the unpleasant task of talking about dying by focusing on clinical details and specific symptoms. Others may be patient and compassionate. Others may be rushed, some are uneasy, and some become coldly detached.

Most of the individuals who shared their experiences were introduced to me because their physicians said they "wouldn't be surprised if the patient died within one year." Although their physicians clearly thought these individuals were "terminally ill," that information was hardly, if ever, communicated to patients in direct, open conversation. Instead, doctors typically talked in a kind of "medical code," which was often only vaguely grasped by patient and families. The purpose of the "coding" was to soften the blow of delivering harsh, devastating news to patients. It also served to protect doctors from having to deal directly with the "big issues" of dying and death.

Delivering bad news is a difficult and unpleasant task, and there are different ways to accomplish it. Some physicians possess the courage and skill to tell the truth while providing reassurance and hope. An internal medicine staff physician provided an example of someone who "softens" bad news and leaves open the possibility for hope. While this physician feels she cannot definitely predict what will happen to any particular patient, she tells patients she thinks are dying that their condition is "serious" or "not good." She warns them that the information she is going to give them is "most important." She tells them "this problem will continue to get worse," but she always gives the "message that there is always something to be done, whether it be pain control, further treatment, or whatever." "I believe in totally telling people the truth, and I think I would say 'this is bad.' But whether or not I would continue to expound on 'this is what's happening, this is the natural progression of this,' I might not do that." This physician rarely uses the words "death" and "dying" in her conversations and tries "very hard to never give time frames." She finds her style "direct" even though patients can clearly interpret the information in a variety of ways.

A few physicians are direct in delivering bad news. One internal medicine resident said that he does not necessarily use the words "death" and "dying"; he relates diagnosis and prognosis to his patients "frankly" but "tactfully." For instance, he might say, "You have a serious condition which may threaten your life, and we don't expect that you will survive it or you will get out of the hospital." This is said along with descriptions of what the patient can expect. For example, he might say, "I think there is an irreversible process that is going on which might lead to eventually your losing your consciousness, going into a coma. You probably might go into a coma." At this point he gauges their reactions. "If they don't believe us, later on maybe we can talk with them again. Not many patients take this well the first time."

It is important to note, however, that communication is not only what doctors say. Medical communication includes the presentation of information by physicians as well as the *processing* of that information by patients and family members. Individual and cultural differences on the patient and family side of the communication are just as varied as are those on the physician side and can cause an identical piece of information delivered in the same manner to be interpreted in completely different ways. Please keep this in mind as you read the story of Mr. Wheeler and the catastrophic miscommunication that took place between him and his doctors. His story not only illustrates poor communication among doctors, patient, and family, it also demonstrates the actual harm that resulted from the "miscommunications" and associated misunderstandings and shows that many patients want information but lack the ability to solicit it from their providers.

As illustrated by the physicians who described this process of giving bad news, cancer treatment options, such as various forms of chemotherapy, surgery, and radiation, as well as the decision-making strategies about when to undergo them, are extremely complicated for anyone to understand. For poor patients with limited education, it is even more difficult. These patients feel intimidated by the medical knowledge of their caregivers. Additionally, they feel disempowered in the medical setting. They are therefore less likely to ask clarifying questions. Most patients are quiet and polite when they meet with their physician, even when they are privately agitated and angry. After the physician leaves the room, however, they often express their confusion, uncertainty, and fear to family members and friends.

Physicians sometimes assess what patients understand about information given by other physicians, but they rarely attempt to obtain feedback on their own delivery of information. One internist confided, "I am much more comfortable asking, 'What did Dr. Lens say, and what do you understand about that?' I ask that question a lot, more than I ask, 'What did I say?' or 'What do you understand about your illness?' " This physician is probably typical in that she assumes her patients understand their illness simply because she explained it. "But how do I know that what I explained made any sense at all?" Occasionally she asks a patient to explain his or her understanding of what she has said, but in general she feels "it was sort of painful to have the conversation the first time, and I'm not sure I want to hear it the second time."

The difficulties of providing full disclosure are multiplied by the fact that the medical element of diagnosis is not always clear and takes some time to determine. In addition, the best course of treatment may not always be readily known and is often subject to debate. Thus, the seriousness of the disease must be communicated at the same time treatment options are explained.

In oncology, for example, this often means the patient must decide whether to undergo the rigors of chemotherapy or other treatments without knowing the exact nature of his or her disease. According to an oncologist, patients should determine whether chemotherapy is "worth it" by balancing symptoms of cancer against symptoms caused by chemotherapy. He uses the metaphor of a balance or an equation. "I tell them I want them to think about all the bad things the cancer is doing to them and put some sort of measure on it." These cancer symptoms are on one side of the equation. On the other side are both the positive and negative effects of the chemotherapy. "On the chemotherapy side, we're going to see if the positive effect of the chemotherapy can be of a greater magnitude than the bad effects of the cancer. And then we're going to have to factor into that equation the known bad effects or side effects of the chemotherapy."

In general, this physician thinks it is almost always worth trying one round of chemotherapy "since we can't know beforehand how anybody's tumor is going to respond or how strong the side effects are going to be." The chemotherapy might be successful either because it "cures" cancer or because it reduces some symptoms, thus improving the patient's quality of life.

"If it turns out that their cancer responds very well, and it eliminates their symptoms, makes them feel better, have more energy, the pain goes away, and that the side effects are either not really bad or they are only transiently bad, then it's reasonable to continue." Obviously, this equation does not always work out this way. "If that equation fails for them, and it doesn't overcome those bad symptoms, then we know that answer. Then we can either try a different chemotherapy, or they have the comfort of knowing they gave it the best shot."

This hope that one form or another of chemotherapy might be successful often delays conversations about hospice or palliative care. "If the patient is getting ready to take chemotherapy, I tend to wait to see if they're going to respond, because I tend not to try to introduce hospice care at the time we're trying to introduce the hope of chemotherapy." This physician thinks introducing chemotherapy and hospice at the same time sends a mixed message, and "they don't understand why we're giving them some hope by treating them, but at the same time putting them in a hospice to die." After several visits, however, the medical team may "evolve a better understanding of their disease and disease progression, and we try to introduce hospice as a means of providing the kind of care that they will likely need and benefit from." This kind of reasoning may be perfectly reasonable from an oncology standpoint, but it makes it more difficult for the patient to come to terms with his or her illness, and more difficult for the medical team and the patient to know what kinds of hopes are reasonable or beneficial, and more difficult to make the decision not to prolong or extend treatment. It also results in hospice referrals being made extremely late in the process, thereby depriving patients and families of important supportive services.

Physicians' perceptions of medical uncertainty make decisions about what to tell patients about their impending deaths, and when, very difficult. An internal medicine physician does not like to talk about when death is expected because she feels that patients are uncomfortable with this subject. As you read the narratives of Mr. White, Mrs. Angel, Mr. Green, Ms. Dickens, and Mr. Noble and witness the steady courage with which they confronted death, it is fair to wonder whether this doctor (and many others) is projecting her uneasiness and fears onto patients. More important for this doctor, however, is that she feels "uncertain" or "insecure" about the prognosis herself. "I think that prognosis is so difficult to predict, and many of the deaths my patients have are fairly acute, unexpected events. But when I know, I will say that when we look at other people like you who have this illness, this is what I think is going to happen. So I try to give the best kind of prognostic stuff that I can, but I am much better at that when patients ask."

In my experience, oncologists, in particular, were extraordinarily accurate in estimating remaining lifespan, but all physicians have stories of patients who lived much longer than was normal with their disease process. They are therefore unlikely to be very direct with their patients about prognosis, sometimes even resisting patient preferences for it. This is especially critical in caring for poor patients, who are less likely to question their doctors assertively. As I will show, the result is that many patients worry about what they are not being told and resent the uncertainty with which they live, becoming privately irritable with their doctors. It should also be noted that none of the physicians asked patients up front how much clinical detail and prognostic information they wanted. Instead, they offered information in

degrees and in styles with which they were most comfortable. The overall consequence for many patients was that they wished their doctors would be more complete and comprehensive in communicating with them.

As discussed in Chapter 2, sustaining hope is an important part of the process of
confronting one's mortality. Among physicians there is real respect for how the powers of hopelessness and hope affect the dying process. This respect causes physicians
to fear being too explicit or pessimistic in the presentations of their findings. Hope
can keep patients showing up at the clinic, whereas if they are in despair and think
nothing can be done they may not come and may miss out on the often beneficial effects of palliative therapies. Unfortunately, however, in this frame of medical thinking, hope is too often confused with curative treatment as opposed to quality of life
and, perhaps, quality of dying, both of which may be enhanced by earlier referrals to
palliative care and hospice. Providers fear that some patients will literally "go home
to die" after they are given a specific terminal prognosis that dashes hope. Physicians
also believe that a poor prognosis that is outlived can damage the doctor–patient relationship. "There are definitely those people who have heard that they have three
months to live so they go home and they sit, waiting for the three months. And then
they get pissed off when they are still alive at four months or five months."

In addition, physicians respect the role hope plays in the final stages of life, particularly hope that is treatment based, even if it seems unreasonable in medical
terms. They feel presumptuous attempting to discount that hope. "I have never
tried to discourage any hope from anybody. At that point in the journey of a
chronic illness that's going to lead to death, I have no problem with whatever a person wants to cling to. As long as it doesn't consume their bank account."

Two examples will suffice to demonstrate the complexity of delivering prognostic information in the context of medical uncertainty. When Bill Wheeler first met
his oncologist, the location of his tumor had not yet been determined. Therefore,
he received a "catch-all" diagnosis of "carcinoma of unknown primary." In this
particular medical center, fifteen percent of people with cancer receive this diagnosis. As a group these people do very poorly, although over the last several years
certain combinations of drugs have been found to benefit a minority of them.
Mr. Wheeler's physician thought he would die within the year, and he introduced
me to him, thinking he would be a good participant for my project. However, if
Mr. Wheeler was one of the rare, fortunate ones who responded to these medications, it was possible that he would not die so quickly. Because the oncologist at that
point judged Mr. Wheeler to be in "reasonable" health, he felt that "it would not be
unrealistic to try one or two cycles of chemotherapy."

After Mr. Wheeler received his first course of chemotherapy, he came to the
clinic and was examined by the fellow in charge of his care. He felt very sick and
nauseated and had lost a great deal of weight. However, his tumor showed signs of
responding to the chemotherapy. The fellow wanted to convey to Mr. Wheeler that
he was not doing well, but he knew that he was unsuccessful in his attempt. "I did

not really press very hard in order to tell him what was wrong because I thought the only thing that was going for him is that he was holding on to some hope. I had no objective basis other than a little weight loss to tell him that his disease was progressing. . . . I didn't want to destroy his last hope." Clearly, this physician was unwilling to push Mr. Wheeler to accept the clinical reality of his disease, particularly in light of the potential benefit of his hopefulness, even if it was rooted in denial. The physician added, "Looking at his overall disease, the fact that he fought prolonged his life. He should have been dead two months ago." It is critical to keep this provider's perspective in mind when reading Mr. Wheeler's account of their interaction, as the difference between their narratives is illustrative of a serious problem in the care of many dying patients. In fact, after their discussion Mr. Wheeler came to believe that not only was the tumor responding to treatment but also that things were looking good and that he would get well again. This was exactly the opposite of what the doctor knew but failed to successfully communicate.

Another patient with diagnostic and prognostic uncertainty was Mrs. Angel. She had a prior history of head and neck cancer that was successfully treated, then subsequently was found to have masses in her lung and a painful swelling in her neck. When the oncologist first met her, clinical evaluation suggested that this could be either her head and neck cancer recurring or a new lung cancer. New cancers are not unusual in someone with a long smoking history "because everyplace tobacco smoke goes, those tissues are at risk to become cancerous."

This medical uncertainty made the discussion of treatment options and prognosis very difficult. "We talked to her about this dilemma of whether this cancer was a recurrence from her head and neck or a brand new lung cancer, and that the treatment for those would use two distinctly different chemotherapy regimens, and at that point I don't think we had a discussion yet about the likely inevitability of it being a terminal event." Based on their best judgment and clinical experience, they designed her chemotherapy as if it were head and neck cancer coming back. "But it didn't work, and in fact her tumor grew a little bit." Her physician therefore recommended stopping that chemotherapy and trying a different one. "Both she and her daughter were very upset by the fact that it didn't work, and so my emphasis at that point was to say, 'Well, there's still hope left because I'm going to take that to mean that it wasn't your head and neck cancer coming back, but it's a totally different cancer, and let's try to change the chemotherapy regimen and see if we get a response.'" Although he was trying to communicate to her that there was still hope, her anxious and tearful response led him to conclude that "she felt that everything had failed. And that could have been that I tried to give her too much information in too little time, or that I didn't try to assess her understanding of that, whatever reason, I think that she had felt that all her hope had been taken away."

Throughout this complex navigation among diagnosis, prognosis, and hope runs the patients' task of setting goals and continuing to live during the dying process. Ideally, the purpose of giving patients "clear and complete information" is so they can make health-care and life decisions that accord most closely with their values. Physicians who often work with dying patients consider helping patients set these goals to be part of their professional responsibility, and patients' goals, in fact, should help determine what kind of medical treatment is appropriate.

An oncologist explained, "I try to be as explicit as I can, and at the same time offer out the possibility that along that path . . . there are many things that can be considered victories, and then we tend to go through that." He offered an example that was fresh in his mind. He had had a second meeting with a patient who was participating in a clinical trial and was scheduled to begin chemotherapy the following day. The patient indicated that he was reluctant to take chemotherapy because of the side effects, and he wanted to know what would happen if he did not take chemotherapy. The physician said the cancer would continue to grow and would give him the kinds of side effects that a cancer in the lung creates, such as shortness of breath and pain. Then the patient said, "And, like death."

That conversation then became the catalyst to discuss the patient's goals. The patient indicated that he never wanted to be dependent on anyone and wanted to remain independent and live alone. "And so as I discussed chemotherapy with him . . . and the value of independent time, I tried to discuss that in terms of: it's possible that the chemotherapy would give him more independent time than not taking chemotherapy." In this case the patient and physician agreed about the prognosis and worked together to set meaningful goals "that may make his death better for him." His acceptance of chemotherapy might lead to a victory in terms of giving him additional independent time, even if it did not significantly shrink his tumor. "So we tried to create a dynamic balance between what, in fact, is inevitable as the disease progresses and what things along the way can be considered as victorious to what an individual patient wants."

Goals must be drastically reconceived when a treatment fails. An oncologist told the story of a woman with a form of lung cancer that a "small but real" number of people beat. "She was a year and a half out, and she and her husband had decided that they had beat it, and they were going to take a humongous vacation. It was their dream." On the last clinic visit before this vacation, she had a chest X-ray that showed her cancer had come back. "And I can remember looking at the chest X-ray, and my heart just sank, and I had to sit down for a while to get ready, because they literally had their tickets, you know, in their hand. I recall sitting down for a minute just to get ready to go into the room. But that was the end of their dream." Goals were reassessed and changed, and they found "victory in that they were able to celebrate a fortieth wedding anniversary at home, and we made it our goal that she was going to be alive for that. They had a huge celebration with family and friends, and it was a joyous occasion. She died shortly after that."

Some goals, however, are not amenable to change and lead to a sense that some deaths are more tragic than are others because there is no way to find meaning in the last stages of life. "I can remember a guy in his mid- to late twenties, a black guy who had just a terrible kind of cancer. No chemotherapy worked with him, not a single thing. He came to clinic one day, and he said that every man needed to make his mark, and that he felt that he was not going to." His physician found this situation "just extraordinarily sad because he truly aspired to lifting himself up and accomplishing something." His physician tried to help this young man find a meaningful path through the dying process but was unsuccessful. "We tried to talk just as person to person, not as doctor to patient, about how you can make a mark, how many different ways a person can make marks. That really never took because he, out of the frustration of dying young, dropped out of our clinic system and had some unfortunate accidents, and came back at a time when he was very close to dying." Unfortunately, as is the case for many of the dying poor, hospice care was arranged for him at the very last moment.

What we have learned so far is that physicians have very different communication styles and bring very different background assumptions to their patient encounters. However, there are some similarities that affect the ways in which doctors care for dying patients. All physicians want to give clear medical information while still allowing for individual variations in disease course and prognosis, both to accommodate clinical ambiguity and the patient's hope. According to these physicians and in my own observations, doctors sometimes live up to their own ideals. Sometimes they do not.

Even their ideals may have some adverse consequences for patients. The ways in which physicians respond to diagnostic and prognostic uncertainty is understandable, although it has two potentially negative effects for patients. First, the information is given in such a vague way that it allows patients to draw virtually any conclusion they want about the future course of their illnesses. Patients I observed generally assumed the most positive interpretation of vague or complex medical information, and they were generally bitter when they turned out to be sicker than they had thought. This dynamic poisons the doctor–patient relationship at a time when it may be most important.

The second potential problem with physician unwillingness to be forthcoming about prognosis is delayed hospice or palliative care referral. Most physicians, especially oncologists, do not think it makes sense to begin discussions about hospice care as long as there is hope of improvement or a treatment that can still be tried, even if survival is really not expected.

Throughout my partnership with patients, I was able to see at least a little of what they saw during a visit with their physicians. Not surprisingly, I found that patients responded to physicians who were kind to them and made an effort to personalize their relationships or even visit them in their homes. Ask patients at County what makes a good doctor, and they will respond "one who listens and acts like a friend." Of course, this relationship, or bond, was possible only when the patient saw the same physician more than once. The assumption of good motives and a caring attitude seemed to be one of the most important factors in how patients felt about their physicians, regardless of the kind of information or technical care they received.

Occasionally, a patient's and family's trust and appreciation exceed the physician's own assessment of his or her work, and this causes special pain for the practitioner. One physician told about one of her patients who had died the previous year of colon cancer. "He had been my patient, and I really felt like it had been my responsibility to make that diagnosis. And I didn't make that diagnosis until it was quite advanced." In her mind, her medical failure was compounded by her neglect to refer the patient to hospice. "Somehow, his wife arranged hospice care. I think a friend must have told her that she needed to call the hospice, and she did. And then I made one visit, and you would have just thought that I was the most wonderful person in the world by making a visit to the home after feeling like I really have not done a good job caring for this patient or his family." Her feelings of inadequacy were compounded by the warm and thankful response she got from the man's wife. "She wrote me just a wonderful 'thank you' note, and she was so grateful that I came to the house. But, in fact, I felt terribly responsible for his death and very badly about not doing earlier hospice care. Fortunately, she took care of her husband."

The strengths and weaknesses of the public hospital system affect those who die within its care to different degrees and in different ways. For some, CHS played a small but significant role. For them it was both a place where they received comfort and caring as well as a place of confusion and hassle, but in the end other factors, such as faith and family, took center stage in their dying processes. For others their experiences in CHS loomed as one of the most important issues in their experiences of dying. They came to the system with a sense of anger or mistrust, often interpreting chaos as purposeful neglect and uncertainty as malicious miscommunication. Thus, the enigmatic system that is the public hospital is one component that shapes the lives of the urban dying poor. I turn now to their stories, keeping in mind how the ideals of caring practitioners, as expressed in this chapter, translate into realities of experience for patients and families, while also exploring myriad other factors that shape the quality of their lives and deaths.

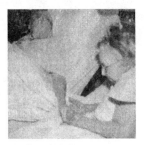

Chapter

4

COURAGE THROUGH
SUFFERING: SNAPSHOTS
OF THE DYING POOR

This chapter revolves around four unique narratives: the Whites, Ms. Annie Dickens, Mr. J. W. Green, and Mr. Joe Noble. The narrative of the Whites vividly depicts the impact of poverty on the dying experience. Despite having worked regularly throughout his life, Mr. White's income was barely sufficient to meet the needs of the family. Together, he and his wife struggled to make ends meet and successfully raise their children. The financial demands they faced each week never allowed them to plan for the future or get ahead in life. As a result, poverty played a significant part in their dying experiences, fostering indignity and exacerbating suffering. Despite being poor, the experience of dying for Ms. Annie Dickens was different. In the very same nursing home where Mr. and Mrs. White endured regrettable indignities, Annie died peacefully and appreciatively. Her faith was a constant source of solace and strength that enabled her to relate to others joyfully and gratefully. The chronicle of Mr. Green's experience of dying demonstrates the consequences of urban and rural poverty. The power of faith is also evident, and in the face of major chaos and conflict in his family life, it gave transcendent meaning throughout his dying. For Mr. Joe Noble, spirituality was not expressed in formal connection to established religious practices. Instead, it was a reflection of the way he lived. He found purpose and meaning in family relationships and in nature. His joy and love of life were derived from these and provided enduring strength throughout enormous physical torment. In these stories, the portraits of dying in inner-city poverty will be richly portrayed, its complexities, triumphs, and difficulties illuminated along with the interwoven dynamics of suffering, financial worry, anger, mistrust, faithfulness, gratitude, family conflict, and family support.

In Shakespeare's *King Lear* there is a scene in which the king and his two retainers encounter a naked beggar. The old king looks first at himself, then at the naked man, and says:

> Ha.
> Here's three on's are sophisticated!
> Thou art the thing itself.

Like the king's robes, there can be snobbery and elitism in academic writing. Intellectual activity, although interesting and important, is often pretentious and removed from the real lives of ordinary people. Like the naked beggar, however, the thing itself is the experience of the suffering human beings that inhabit the world of the dying poor. In order to honor their lives, their stories must assume center stage. Thus, in this chapter and in those that follow, I return to people. The goal is to let their stories speak for themselves. When observation and analyses enter the narrative, it is only secondary to their experiences and for the express purpose of helping to explain what I saw in their lives on a regular basis, so others may come to know them better.

The Injuries of Poverty:
Mr. and Mrs. White

> Tell me you think he wasn't rude.
>
> —Ken White

Like so many of the inner-city indigent, Ken and Virble White lived in ways that destroy the prevailing stereotypes in which the poor are portrayed. Neither lazy nor irresponsible, the Whites were salt-of-the-earth people. They were in a stable, loving marriage of forty-three years. Virble raised their four children while Ken worked all his life to support their family. He toiled hard, often doing unpleasant and difficult work. He was always able to provide for his family even if only at a minimum level. For the last twenty-nine years of his life he worked at a wholesale fish market that served most of the restaurants and food stores in Indianapolis. Ken told the story:

> I worked there twenty-nine years. I worked for twenty-five years and retired. I went home and sat around the house there. Took a little trip to Topeka, Kansas, and came back. . . . Then I went back to work. I went back four years, and, of course, I was retired, so I could only make eight thousand a year.

When describing the work that he did, Mr. White talked about it most matter-of-factly:

> Sometimes in the winter, when you had a wind chill of 30° below zero, there were a lot of times I had to work outside for an hour or two. What I would do is go out there and work until I felt myself getting chills, then I would pour a shot of whiskey and a cup of coffee and get back to work. That was the one thing the boss did not allow. The boss does not allow anyone to drink on the job, so I sneaked it when I was taking inventory.

In describing some of his other responsibilities he recalled how, "I also had to clean the shithouse, because of the board of health. You would not believe how dirty these sewers can get. You wouldn't believe what it is, how not clean at all."

This job, which he held for twenty-nine years, paid enough money that he could afford his rent, buy groceries, pay the insurance on the clunker car he drove, buy clothes from the local discount store, and have a little left over for beer on the weekend. It provided neither health insurance nor a pension. It did, however, enable Ken, Virble, and their children to live week to week and month to month. In this situation they faced unrelenting financial pressure and hardship. It seems very ironic that while much of the

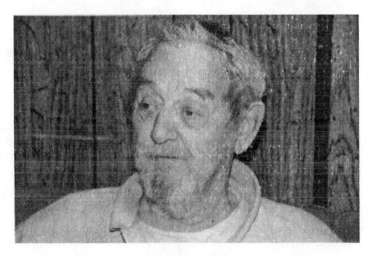

"I'm Catholic, you know," said Ken during our first conversation together. His faith would become his major source of guidance throughout dying.

nation was basking in unprecedented prosperity, Ken and Virble, like many other "invisible Americans," were struggling to get by. Their rental house was in a dingy, deteriorating, and marginally safe neighborhood. Its interior was cluttered, slightly dirty, and, like many of the houses of inner-city patients, dark. The Whites severely restricted the use of their lights for financial reasons. A console TV, a velvet recliner, and decorative plates in a china cabinet were their prized possessions. The television served a dual function: it provided cheap entertainment and helped to light the house. Nonetheless, despite a lifetime of economic struggle, they lived joyfully and meaningfully together for forty-three years.

I first met Mr. White in February 2000, exactly one week after he had been diagnosed with esophageal cancer. The diagnosis quickly brought havoc into his life. Without knowing all the medical details, he instinctively knew how serious his situation was. His anxiety in receiving such bad news was compounded by the fact that he was the primary caretaker of his beloved wife. Ten years his senior and debilitated from chronic lung disease, Mrs. White was unable to care for herself. She needed help to get from bed to a chair, lacked the strength to toilet herself, and was utterly dependent on him to perform all the household chores, which he did dutifully and gladly, rarely complaining. Thus, his diagnosis was huge not just in terms of its implications for him but for his wife and her future as well.

He knew that this was a time in life for choices—hard choices. First, he was going to have to make decisions about his medical care. Second, he needed to come up with a plan to ensure that his wife would be cared for. Caring for her had become increasingly difficult in recent months. He had suffered a heart attack the preceding December, and now with the cancer diagnosis he knew things were only going to get worse. Third, he worried about their forty-year-old son, Danny, who was living with them. Danny had suffered a stroke within the past year, and his ability to care for himself was impaired by stroke-related deficits. Mr. White pondered over how he might ensure that Danny would be taken care of.

He resolved the first situation quickly. He had seemed to have made up his mind that he was not going to have chemotherapy even before I met him. "I'm Catholic, you know, and if this is God's will, then that's that," he said with thoughtfulness. He seemed fairly certain about this decision but decided not to shut the door completely on treatment until he heard what the oncologist had to say. His appointment was scheduled the following week, and he would wait until then to make a final determination.

When the day of his appointment arrived, Danny dropped Mr. White off at the hospital. He went to the oncology clinic to check in, and the unit secretary told him that he had a $25 co-payment. Mr. White told her honestly, "I don't have $25, but I have an appointment to see the doctor." The secretary told him there was nothing she could do and that he would have to get the matter straightened out with the financial services office. Irritated, Mr. White left the desk and went in search of financial services. Lost and dizzy after wandering around for about ten minutes, he was escorted to the office by a volunteer who noticed his disorientation. Once there, he discovered that the financial information that made him eligible for the "indigent program" had somehow been deleted from the computer system. The person in financial services got him recertified, and thirty minutes later he was headed back to the oncology clinic, annoyed and not feeling well. There, he waited well beyond his scheduled appointment time to see the oncologist.

The oncology fellow came in and explained the course of treatment that his cancer would require. Mr. White listened to the entire presentation and then told the doctor that he was not going to opt for chemotherapy. "On hearing me say that, he got abrupt, rude, real rude, and got up and left." A bit later in our conversation, he went on to reaffirm his experience. "Yeah, he was rude. Not that I give a shit." Clearly, his words and the tone in which they were spoken demonstrated that he cared very much about this doctor's attitude. He talked about it often in subsequent conversations, feeling that his doctors did not give him the respect he deserved. As a result, Ken left the oncology clinic that day with a bit of an attitude. Upon checking out with the unit secretary, he was given a slip of paper with a return appointment in two months.

Although I hesitate to disrupt the narrative at this point, an important issue must be addressed. Instead of being sent home with a return appointment, an appointment that truly

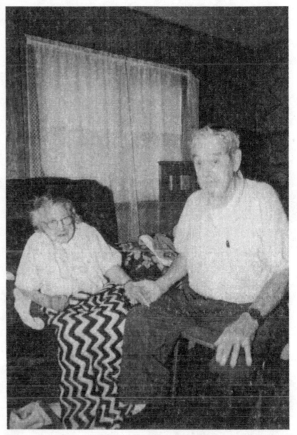

Ken and Virble married on June 14, 1956, and remained married for forty-three years. "He can park his shoes under my bed anytime," Virble said to her mother after her first date with Ken.

seemed useless given his expressed wish not to begin treatment, another approach would have been more appropriate. It would have been more valuable for the oncologist to say something such as, "Well, Mr. White, while I disagree with your decision, I respect your right to make it. Since you have decided against treatment, let me tell you about another option that might interest you. Have you heard of hospice or palliative care?"

I raise this point to emphasize that Mr. White's experience is reflective of a national problem. In our death-avoiding culture with its focus is on aggressive curative treatment, far too many dying persons are never referred to hospice, or if they are, the referral is made extremely late in the course of illness. On a national level, the problem is one of zealous overuse and timid underuse, that is to say, overuse of sophisticated technology and underuse of measures that will reduce suffering. In this framework, concern for comfort and quality of life are deferred in preference to technological interventions. For the urban poor, especially African Americans, the problem is even more acute. As discussed in Chapter 2, feelings of disempowerment combined with widespread mistrust leave patients and families uncertain and suspicious about hospice and palliative care. In this frame of mind they are reluctant to shift gears away from curative treatment. Often those options, when cure is not the goal, are seen as another form of deprivation among a population that already feels medically, economically, and socially deprived.

One week after his oncology appointment, Mr. White became extremely lightheaded and dizzy. Immediately, 911 was called, and he was rushed to the emergency room (ER). His blood sugar was severely elevated, 1,200 to be precise, and he had a urinary tract infection. After getting him stabilized, the ER doctor joked with him. "You were the walking dead, my friend. When your sugar reached 700, you should have passed out." To ensure that his blood sugar would remain stabilized, Ken was admitted into the hospital, where he continued to complain bitterly about the earlier incident in the oncology clinic. "Tell me you think he wasn't rude," he said, going on to exclaim

> He went yak, yak, yak, yak. All I said was fine, fine. He then said we will go into chemotherapy and we will cut some of the cancer out. And I said not for one damn second. And he got up and left.

He continued:

> Well, the minute he gets up and walks out because I told him I am not going through chemotherapy, I would say that is pretty rude. And I just got a referral slip in the mail for another appointment. Can you believe that? I threw it away. I wasn't about to go back and talk to him, because I'm not having any therapy or any cutting. They cannot seem to get it through their minds that I'm not going to have it. They better, though, because I don't want them to waste my time or theirs.

These are strong words, indeed, words indicative of the fact that Mr. White, while angry at the oncologist, was firm in his decision not to proceed with treatment. This decision, morally and legally his to make, was made comfortable for him by his faith in God.

> Now, there is one thing about these doctors, they all want to cut on me and give me chemotherapy and all of this other stuff. And I

absolutely refuse any such treatment. I've lived this long. I've lived
for seventy-one years with this, not with the terminally ill part,
but I've lived for seventy-one years. I am going to die. God is going
to take me to a new life when it is time for me to go, not before,
and that's the way I feel about it. I've been hurt several times.
Could have been dead a couple of times. I'm still here, so apparently God has some use for me yet. Until he doesn't, no cutting!

I should interject at this point that given the extent to which his disease had progressed, the oncologists had little to offer. Perhaps they were disinclined to refer
him to hospice because of their stated belief that every patient should go through
"at least one or two rounds of chemotherapy." The medical reality, however, was
that no treatment could cure the disease, significantly extend his life, or likely improve his quality of life. In fact, when one of the primary care doctors heard about
what had happened, he snapped, "Do you know what they have to offer him?" An-
swering his own question, he exclaimed, "Nothing!" Consequently, this doctor
took it upon himself to contact Mr. White and inquire if he would be interested in
a referral to hospice and palliative care. It was in this round-about way that Ken
and Virble made their way into palliative care and eventually hospice.

Ken proceeded to talk about being steadfast in his decision with calm and serenity. His tone of voice softened as he said,

I am very comfortable with my decision. I am a Catholic and was
born a Catholic; I was baptized in the church seventy-one years
ago. I believe in God's ways. If we Catholics can't do it, nobody
can. Either you go when he tells you, or you are not going to go to
heaven. That's the way I believe it. And that's the way I believed it
for seventy-one years, and will continue to believe it until I die.

Thus, faith was the basis on which Mr. White came to his decision. It was also a
source of strength and consolation that enabled him to maintain a bright outlook,
despite the enormous suffering that had afflicted his life over the past several years.
Ken had much with which to cope. His wife's illness progressed to the point that
she was essentially bed ridden. A year before his diagnosis his son Dean had died
from a stroke. Ken and Virble walked into his house and found him dead on the living room floor, his head held in the lap of his wife. As you will recall, their other
son, Danny, had suffered a stroke just ten months before. Additionally, before receiving his cancer diagnosis, Ken had gotten diabetes and had had a heart attack. It
cannot be forgotten that all these experiences of illness, loss, and grief took place
within the context of persistent financial hardship. It is not melodramatic to state
that Ken and Virble knew suffering as a close companion, especially during the few
preceding years. Nevertheless, like so many of the dying poor, Ken spoke about
these tribulations with a remarkable sense of tolerance:

It really hasn't been really all that bad. I haven't had too much trouble with it, except my health had been a lot better than what it is. My health has went down hill in the last few months. I had my heart attack in December. My health has gotten to a point where I don't have control over anything. I can't get up. I can't move. I can't get around.

When asked how he was able to cope with all he had faced recently, he reiterated, "I'm okay, it really isn't so bad," and that he placed God at the center of his life. Believing that poverty, illness, grief, and death was "a test of my faith," Mr. White prayed regularly. "Just general prayer," he noted. "I am not asking for anything. If he wants me, he's going to take me." In conversations with him, I asked if dying frightened him, and he responded with calm and certainty. "Not in the slightest. Why should it? What is it?" Without pausing, he went on to remark:

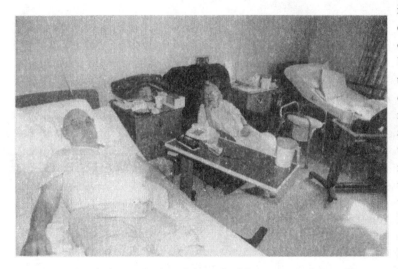

Husband and wife facing death and the end of their relationship in the nursing home.

Well, it's going to sleep and not waking up. Death is just a continuation of sleep. Sometimes I think that is all it is. The body dies but the mind and spirit do not. I don't think the mind ever does. I guess I'm funny in some ways. I just don't believe all of that. You go to heaven or hell, and you are going to go when it's your time, and you are going to go when God tells you you're going to go.

It is remarkable how quickly Mr. White came to terms with dying. Although angry at some of the care he received, an anger that would only intensify as he got sicker and endured more disrespectful treatment, he was at peace with his personal fate. Correspondingly, he remained at peace with his decision not to pursue treatment for his cancer.

Having dealt with these matters swiftly and to the point of equanimity, he then turned his attention to his wife and her needs. He had made up his mind that a nursing home was the only workable option for them. Virble was initially resistant to the idea, having earlier had a bad experience as a patient in a nursing home. Reluctantly, she agreed to go to Deerfield Village, saying, "We've been together for forty-three years, I can't leave him now." So, in a fog of depression that stayed with her throughout her stay, she relocated to the nursing home.

From the beginning, their experience was unpleasant. Most significant was the "excremental assault" they experienced as a consequence of neither sheets being changed nor bedside toilet being emptied regularly. The sad fact of the matter was that most of the time their room had a foul order from urine and feces. The problems began the first weekend they spent in the nursing home. As Mr. White bitterly explained on the following Monday,

> Well, you ask me how things are going, and, you know me, I have to tell it straight out. . . . She shat her pants and was forced to lay in it, because I couldn't help her, you know.

Asked to elaborate, he continued:

> Well, she shit herself. I'm waiting for the nurse to come in, so they can help her out and get her cleaned up and everything. And they said the nurse couldn't help her. That she was pregnant and couldn't lift her up or anything. She said she'd get some help in here. And I guess about thirty, thirty-five minutes later I rang for the nurse again. Nobody ever showed up. About thirty, thirty-five minutes I rang for the nurse again. Nobody showed up. She has been laying in shit all this time. About an hour later, an aide came in to give her some medicine, and I told her about it. She has been laying there in that bed for over two hours, laying there in her own shit before she got changed or cleaned up or anything. Now that is treatment that I don't think is right in no way, shape, or form.

Later, he told of other episodes:

> Well, she peed several times and had to lay in it quite a while before they came in and changed her. I helped her up a while ago and got her on the pot . . . of course she can't control herself whatsoever.

One morning, before I could even greet him and say hello, he blurted out,

> It happened again. This time she laid in her own shit for seven hours!

He went on to explain that she awoke around 4:30 AM on a Sunday morning with stomach discomfort. She had a bowel movement in the bed at 5:00, and it took until noon to get her cleaned, changed, and back into bed with fresh linens. As one might imagine, his anger was increasing with each incident, which created a tension between him and the staff that only made the situation worse. Ironically, when asked if he ever spoke to anyone about the horrendous care Virble was getting, he replied,

> No, I didn't say too much. I know that they have a lot of people to take care of, but they still shouldn't have someone lay like that.

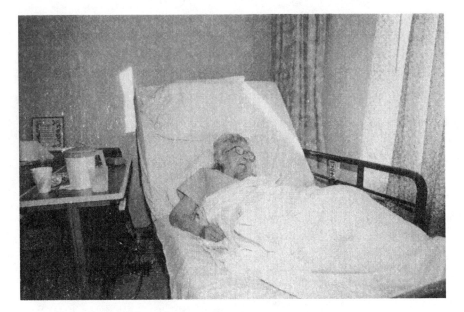

Prozac did nothing to comfort or console.

As Mr. White became sicker and unable to toilet himself, he encountered the same problem. He would lie in urine-soaked sheets while Virble helplessly looked on. Never having the strength or empowerment to complain directly to the nursing home staff, she would quietly express her pain in whispered tones: "You know those nurses don't have to get so rough with Kenny when he wets the bed. He can't help it." She further revealed, "It is so hard to watch him lay there like that."

Having no other option available to them, the Whites were stuck in the nursing home, and, being poor, they were stuck in this particular one. Their days were long, and visitors were few. A nun would come weekly and give religious instruction to Virble, who was converting to Catholicism. A priest or Eucharistic minister would come to administer Communion on Friday afternoon. Most of the day Ken would watch TV on the console they brought from home. Virble would stare out the window or gaze lovingly at him. She was becoming increasingly listless. Her doctor prescribed Prozac, but it did very little to alleviate her depression. Day after day their facial expressions told the story of how deeply they were suffering and how unimaginably difficult it was to be facing separation from a forty-three-year-long relationship.

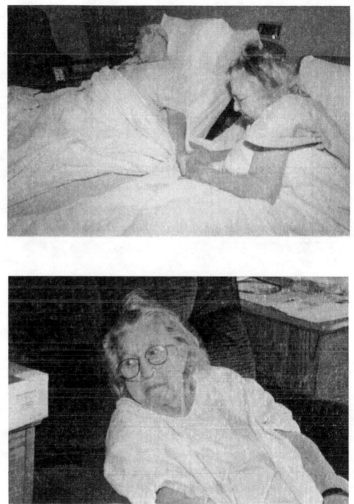

After three months in Deerfield Village, it was becoming clear that Mr. White was going to die first. Virble, without anyone telling her, sensed that his death was approaching and began worrying about the future. "I don't know where I'm going. Linda tells me that I can't go back home as we've lost the house." By statute,

The pain of anticipating the death of a spouse.

after sixty days in Deerfield Village the Whites' social security income, which paid their rent, had been diverted to the nursing home. As a result, they would be formally evicted in another thirty days. She also worried about Danny. Although he was an infrequent visitor, she knew he was going to have a difficult time making it on his own, and she worried intensely about Kenny's funeral. During an especially striking conversation, she asked if

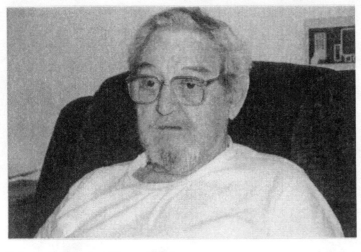

"I hope she dies first," he confided.

I "might be able to get Kenny a suit so he could be buried in it. He doesn't have many clothes. He usually wears a T-shirt around the house or a work shirt, but he doesn't have any dress clothes." I found it particularly poignant that she expressed no humiliation while asking for help. In a life of poverty, such financial urgency was a matter of daily experience. She trusted me and other members of the palliative care team and was therefore comfortable making this request. For several weeks she incessantly worried that she could not arrange a proper funeral and that Kenny would have to endure one more "final indignity."

In the last ten days of his life, Ken became less livid, and his anger waned. By choice or otherwise, he was submitting to the imperatives of his disease-ridden body. His pain was minimal, but the care he got—whether it was being toileted or fed or receiving medication—remained inconsistent. His wife would look on passively when things did not go right for him. This was an unimaginably difficult time for her. She watched, powerless, as his body succumbed to the will of the disease, feeling deeply hurt by the indignity of his care, and all along worrying about when "the day will finally come" and "he'll be gone." Wanting to be near him at the end, her bed was pushed over next to his, and they slept side-by-side as husband and wife until he died on a Friday morning.

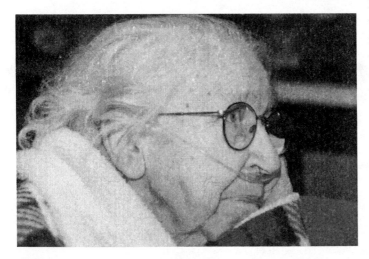

Words cannot adequately describe her loss.

The good news for Virble was that her sixty-year-old daughter decided to take her home the day Ken died. The bad news was that her beloved Kenny was gone, compounded by the fact that she truly did not have the money for his funeral. The body had been picked up by a local funeral home, where it remained un-touched on Friday, Satur-day, Sunday, and Monday. After much effort by the hospice social workers, arrangements were made with the trustees office to pay for "a pauper's funeral" late Tuesday afternoon.

Finally, on Wednesday afternoon, the viewing was held. Mr. White had gotten his suit and his body lay in the cloth-covered, pressed wood casket that is stan-dard fare for a pauper's funeral arranged by the trustees office. Virtually no attention was paid to Mrs. White by the funeral home staff. The indifference to the family was so notice-able that the palliative care team nurse remarked, "I wonder if they treat their paying customers this way?"

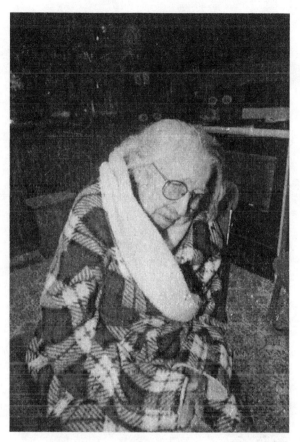

Feelings of helplessness loomed large as Ken's body lay in limbo while the funeral home waited for financial arrange-ments to be made.

After the funeral mass and burial, Mrs. White went home with her daughter Nancy. Nancy had decided that her mother would live with her until she died.

The palliative care team had invited itself into the Whites' lives without referral and had become very close to both of them during the preceding two months. The team made regular home visits. They brought flowers and arranged for a special celebration on the day that would have been their forty-fourth anniversary. Virble chose the menu: Church's fried chicken, green beans, and mashed potatoes. They sat on the front porch, and Virble joked about the buff bodies of the shirtless con-

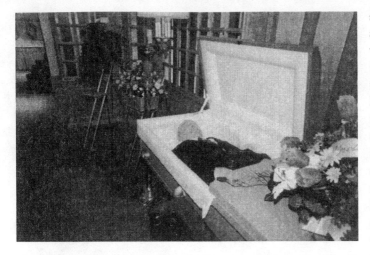

Ken finally got his suit.

struction workers across the street. This was a bittersweet time for her. She suffered through the death of her husband, was getting sicker herself, and worried about Danny. Then, without warning, more tragedy came into her life. Another daughter was rushed to County emergency room with chest pains. She was stabilized and admitted to the coronary care unit, but she did not make it. She died a day later.

It all seemed so odd. The rest of the country was obsessed with who got voted off the island that week, as a prevailing form of "entertainment distraction" during this time was the TV show *Survivor*. Meanwhile Virble White was lying in a hospital bed in her daughter's living room suffering from all that happened during the last year: Ken's illness, Danny's stroke, Dean's death, the indignities of the nursing home, Ken's death, her daughter Helen's death and her own illness, all the while knowing that she was nearing the end of her life. It is absurd that her profound suffering coexisted alongside such a trivial obsession as a TV show. The fact that her suffering was a matter of indifference to so many is striking in its sadness. Despite all these hardships, however, she retained a capacity for joy.

Virble died at home four months after Ken's death. Her daughter lovingly cared for her into her death,

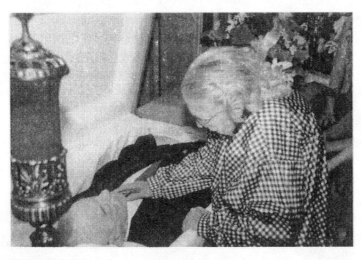

The end of a life and a marriage.

despite the emotional and physical toll it took on her. Unable to afford the funeral, Nancy was also dependent on the trustees office to finance the burial of her mother. Mrs. White's wake was held at the same funeral home as was Ken's. Her funeral service took place at the graveside. It was a "quick and dirty" ceremony that lasted no more than two minutes, at which her name was never even mentioned by the minister, a man who had never met her or the family. Danny, who had stopped off for a pack of cigarettes on the way to the cemetery, missed it entirely.

In sum, there is much in this narrative that is reminiscent of Hawthorne's description of John Treeo. It shows that the sufferings of Ken and Virble were intensified because of their economic and social status, while much of the broader community remained indifferent, yet it also demonstrates a remarkable humanity, strength, and resilience in

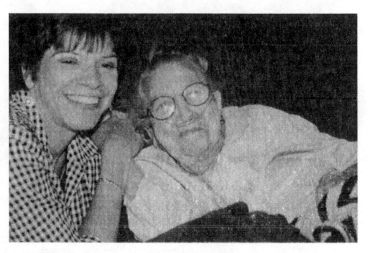

Support and love of the social worker helped see Virble through this difficult time.

the face of severe suffering. I hope that you agree that these "salt-of-the-earth" people deserved better and that as a society we not only could have done better by them, we should have.

Beauty Through Faith While Suffering: Annie Dickens

> I've got to do this for Him.
>
> —Annie Dickens

Upon meeting Annie Dickens for the first time, the words of the poet Yeats sprang to mind. In his poem "Easter" he writes: "He too, has been changed in his turn. Transformed utterly: A terrible beauty is born." While her body was being utterly and hideously transformed by disease, a powerful dignity and grace was emerging. On first sight Annie appeared physically grotesque and revolting. She was emaciated and jaundiced, and her lips were cracked. She labored to speak even the simplest words. In our culture the tendency is to avoid such people. To be in their presence is too difficult, too messy. It elicits pervasive feelings of discomfort about both physical deformity and mortality. Even so, if one were able to penetrate the facade of physical ugliness, one would meet a lovely, striking, and courageous woman. To get to know Annie Dickens, even if just for an hour, was to have had the privilege of witnessing a profile in dignity and courage.

Two years earlier Ms. Dickens had been told she had six months to live. She was living at home at the time and was initially resistant to going to a nursing home. However, getting sicker and less able to care for herself, coupled with the absence of people who could care for her, she was forced into becoming a resident at Deerfield Village. By the time I met her, she had widely progressed lung cancer compounded by chronic lung disease. She had severe shortness of breath and ate virtually nothing. She was on six liters of oxygen per minute and received regular breathing treatments throughout the day. She had extensive peripheral vascular disease and was in a lot of pain, especially when she was moved. On several occasions the oxygen on which her breathing depended had been surreptitiously turned off. It was believed that a roommate, who agonized over how much Annie suffered each day, was responsible. Her intentions presumably were merciful. Nonetheless, she was to be moved to another room on a different floor. After the transfer these incidents never occurred again.

Despite her extensive disease and its crippling impact on her body, Annie never succumbed to depression or sadness. In fact, she would say regularly, "I don't feel sick. I just ask God to take care of me, and that is what He is doing." When asked how she was feeling, invariably her response would be, "I am doing okay." Typically, she would go on to explain that she was thankful. When I inquired what she was grateful for, she said, "I'm grateful for you." Incredible, I thought. Here she was bedridden in a nursing home, and she was grateful for visits from someone who would one day tell a bit of her story. "I'm grateful for Sally," she would add. Sally was one of the volunteers in the palliative care program. She would regularly visit, bringing flowers and her Bible to read. "I am grateful for the care I get here. You know I need to be taken care of. I wasn't able to do it at home. But, let me tell you about what I am most grateful for: God." As Annie struggled to breathe and fought to enunciate the words clearly and loudly enough to be heard, I sat back and listened. This indigent African-American woman, dying in the county nursing home, was becoming my teacher. "There is so much I could tell you," she said. Encouraged to proceed, she continued:

I feel blessed. I really feel that God is taking care of me.

When questioned on how she could feel such peace amid such severity of disease, without hesitating she responded:

I just thank God for life. I know one thing. He don't let me have no pain. Every once and a while I have some pain, when I move, but I just talk to God and thank Him and I don't feel the pain anymore. So, I thank God even though I am very sick, he don't let me have no pain.

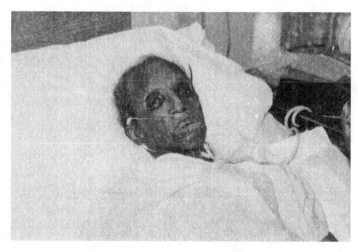

Disease had destroyed her body, but her spirit remained untouchable.

For Annie, God was a soothing balm for infirmity. Through her faith she found purpose and meaning in suffering. "He has a plan for all the things that happen to me," she said with confidence. Conversations with Annie about God were truly stimulating. She reveled in the opportunity to share her faith, reminding me to come back soon so she could tell more. Her faithful spirit was both exhilarating and contagious. Even when she would have a day of particularly severe pain, she never expressed anger but would only say, "I'm hoping tomorrow will be better."

Unlike Mr. White, whose persistent anger was like an undertow dragging him down, Annie's life flowed with gratitude. She continually expressed deep affection for Sally. She would always speak with appreciation about her

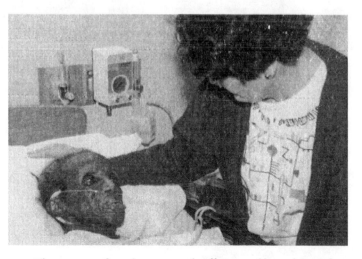

The support of a volunteer eased suffering and brought comfort.

cards, flowers, and prayers, but most of all she was thankful for Sally's compassionate presence in her life. She always greeted her caretakers in the nursing home with a smile and said good-bye with a thank you. On many occasions she would remark, "I'm truly grateful for the people here who take care of me." While Annie was mindful of all these people who cared about and for her, she believed their presence in her life was part of God's plan. "I know one thing, it's God I have to thank. I thank God for putting me in this bed, for if I wasn't here, I wouldn't know where I'd be." Her voice became a bit stronger, and she explained:

> I wasn't able to do it at home, so I thank God. I really truly do, that's no lie. I really thank Him so much for taking care of me. So far He saw fit to put me in this nursing home, so I just thank God for it.

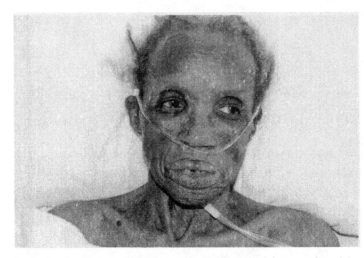

She looked intensely into my eyes and said:

> So very much to thank God for.

Then, peaceful and comfortable as if talking to an old friend, she looked upward. With an almost urgent expression that matched the solemnity of her words, she said:

Body in physical anguish, Annie's spirit and soul are comforted by faith and gratitude.

> Thank you, Jesus. You are the Lord of my life.

For Annie faith was not a theologically abstract entity. Rather, it was a set of beliefs and practices that not only shaped her view of the world but guided her though it. It provided strength and meaning, giving her genuine comfort in the midst of agony. Her words, never contrived, were strong and unwavering:

> I'm not worried. I give it all to Him. I just thank God that I have the comfort that I do, and that is Jesus Christ.

Without missing a beat, Annie began to pray, and I listened intently:

The Lord is my shepherd I shall not want
He leads me to lie down in green pastures
He leads me besides still waters
He restores my soul
My cup runneth over
Surely . . .
All the days of my life and I should live in the house of the Lord.

She struggled to get through the prayer. Her breath was short and labored, and her discomfort was noticeable. Upon finishing she apologized for "not saying it exactly right because I'm getting too forgetful, but that's the part I wanted to say." I responded that it was "just perfect because it came from the heart," to which she replied, "I'm just thankful that He is my shepherd."

It was obvious that Annie's strength came primarily from connectedness to God. "I've got to do this for Him," she affirmed. "He's working it out in his own way. Give it to God and He'll work it

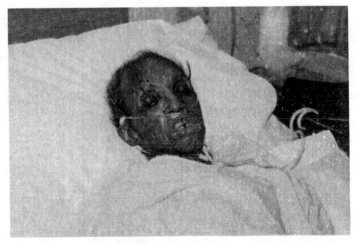

"I give it all to Him," said Annie with purpose.

out. So I'm giving it to God." Annie seemed so majestic, especially in contrast to her body, which was being cannibalized by disease. For those of us who knew her, it was difficult to get her out of our minds. One Thursday afternoon toward the end of a visit, I asked her directly how she was able to face death steadily without fear. Having grown tired and not feeling well, she answered, "Come back on Friday, and I'll tell you." When I saw her the next day, it was obvious that she had worsened significantly. Her breathing was more strained, her pain was elevated, yet she was as gracious as ever, her spirit remaining strong. "Afraid?" she puzzled. "What do I have to be afraid of? The Lord will take me away from here, so, 'Lord I put myself in your hands,'" she said directly to Him, looking up. Turning her attention back to me, she said, "I never think about dying, not really, not seriously. I just say when the Lord gets ready, he will take me. So, I'm not afraid of dying, I'm not worried. Like I say, I give it all to Him."

I then asked Annie how she was able to maintain such an optimistic spirit in the face of very real and relentless physical suffering. When I suggested, "You are having a difficult time here," she agreed, responding, "Yes, I am." She then went on to explain, "I hope things will be better tomorrow. One day at a time. Listen . . . one day at a time." As she struggled for breath, her words became increasingly difficult to understand. Nonetheless, Annie went on to expand on what she meant by "one day at a time":

> I trust in God forever
> Wherever I may be
> On the land, or
> The raging sea.
>
> Come with me,
> I put my trust in Him
> Because he gave me,
> One day at a time.

Annie was so sick at this point that it took nearly two minutes to be able to say these few words. She was determined that I should hear her prayer and patiently repeated herself over and over again so the words could be understood. Annie's Prayer, as I continue to call it, left me speechless. After a few minutes of comfortable silence, I told her, "It is a beautiful prayer," to which she responded immediately, "Yes, it is!"

Before leaving her that day, I told her how much I admired her strength and that she was "just beautiful." Ever grateful, Annie replied, "Thank you." There was a clarity and strength in her voice as she uttered these words, a resonance that she had not been able to achieve for weeks. When I left that day, I did not know that it would be the last time I would see her. Annie died peacefully on a Sunday morning, having profoundly touched the lives of those she knew while a resident in the nursing home. Knowing Annie was a privilege, as is the opportunity to share a part of her story. Thank you, Annie.

Southern Plantation to
Inner-City Streets: J. W.

The rich people don't even know how a poor person lives.
—J. W. Green

Asked about his boyhood memories, J. W. Green responded, "We were poor. Dirt poor. We had nothing at all to play with." These words were spoken in the nursing home in which Mr. Green was dying. Geographically, this nursing home was 1,000 miles from where he grew up. Economically and racially, however, it was similar in many ways. Although an urban environment had replaced the rural setting of his youth, poverty dominated his life from beginning to end. There may have been variations in styles and forms, but economic scarcity shaped his existence from its beginning in rural Mississippi to its end in urban Indianapolis.

On March 17, 1932, Mr. Green was born the twelfth of thirteen children. He was born and raised in a world entirely unfamiliar to most Americans. As he described, "I grew up in Mississippi. It was on a plantation. We were plantation workers and sharecroppers. My dad worked all of his life there, going back to the old-time days." He continued, "Yep, right up by the Mississippi River. This is where we were born and raised at. My mother and father, they lived a whole lifetime together. They got married about 1910. My mother would be about ninety now. My dad, he died at sixty-eight. And my mother died of old age. And, that was unusual under the conditions we were raised up in."

When I inquired what family life was like while growing up, J. W. would always speak about his feeling of closeness to his parents and siblings:

> Yeah, so me and the others are real close. Family has been important the whole life for me. It's been that way all my life. My family is real close.

He elaborated further, with a spirit of pride and confidence strengthening his voice:

> My mother and father were real close, too. We obeyed our parents. We never got too grown to obey mom and dad. That's the way we were raised up. We always raised our brothers and sisters if we could. Family sticks together. Stays together.

Mr. Green spoke often of family, always expressing how important it was to him. Throughout his adult years and into his death, family played a paradoxical role in his life. It was important to him, yet, despite his convictions about "being there for our family," he failed his children miserably as a father. His first marriage, at the age of sixteen, ended quickly. He was able to sustain his second marriage for thirty-nine years, until his wife, tired of his philandering and "running the streets," sought a divorce. As his death approached, he worried that he would die lonely, abandoned by his children as he had abandoned them. In this regard, for the most part, his fears were realized. His children were indifferent to his illness and suffering. Only two of the seven saw him at all during the final six months of his life. But I am getting ahead of myself. I will say more about the dynamics of family support at the end of his life, but first I need to elaborate on his experiences growing up the son of sharecroppers.

J. W. and his family lived poor. Theirs was truly an existence of subsistence. They lived in a shack provided by the owner and were allowed to use a small patch of land to grow vegetables for their own use. They had a small area where they fenced in cows and hogs. Although these animals were raised at the expense of the family, they provided milk to drink and meat to eat. Thus, along with the vegetables that were grown and preserved, there would be enough basic food for the family to survive. In return the Greens had to work in any fashion demanded by the owner. Primarily, J. W.'s family grew cotton on the land owned by "boss man," as they called him. The basic arrangement was that they would be assigned sixty acres on which to plant, chop, and pick cotton. At the end of the day they would be able to keep a percentage of the cotton they picked. The rest belonged to "boss man."

Survival in this life, essentially obsolete in the twenty-first century, was difficult and hard, but not impossible. They sold their portion of the harvested crops, thereby earning enough money for life's necessities. As most of their income was seasonal, "boss man" arranged for credit at the local store, where they would be able to purchase needed goods that they lacked the money to buy otherwise. This arrangement was important to tenant farmers like the Greens, especially during the winter months. These "loans" would be deducted from the next year's wages, which kept the family in a continual state of indebtedness. The family could always count on the loans to be forthcoming, because there was incentive for the owner to ensure that they would have sufficient resources to survive. He needed them to be strong and healthy to work the fields. Ironically, J. W. and his family took all this in stride. It was the only life they knew, and they seemed to live it with a remarkable sense of dignity. As J. W. explained:

> We had a rich life in a lot of ways. We had no money. We had a rich life coming up, though, which was the thing that really took care of us. From our sisters and mother we learned how to make long quilts and clothes. We had a good sewing machine.

Particularly impressive is that while the experience of poverty was always severe, J. W. was neither bitter about nor resentful of his childhood experiences in the South. In fact, he spoke proudly of his home there, especially the connection to the earth and family that he was only "able to feel in Mississippi."

In this subsistence mode of living, J. W.'s mother and father were never able to get ahead. With the birth of each child, they could not even remain economically stable but rather were pulled backwards. Thus, for J. W. poverty was

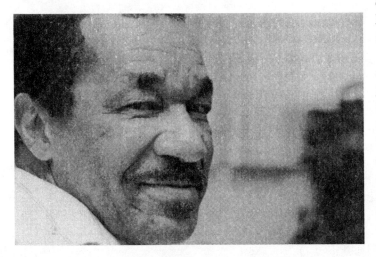

J. W. reminisces about life as a sharecropper in Mississippi.

historic, that is to say, it was inherited and transmitted by his heritage. He recognized the stark fact that unless he made a move, his life would not just be like his parents', it would be even more economically desperate. So, this young man, who truly lived, breathed, and bled a life of agricultural poverty, migrated to a Midwestern city:

> I left there when I was twenty-five. I've been here ever since. And I'm sixty-six now. I left my mother and father. I was the last kid to leave home when I was grown up. I was twenty-five years of age. I was looking for a bit of life for my family. The first four years I was married, I couldn't be the father of two children with the money I was making there. Back then it was every man for himself, you know, the farmers. And we weren't getting but $4.50 a day for work. That was in '56.

Displaced from his roots, J. W. came to the city as an uneducated black man whose farming skills were not marketable in the urban environment. He worked at odd jobs, but, faced with racial discrimination and genuine lack of opportunity, he turned to the streets for his livelihood and entertainment. Ironically, J. W. had come to Indianapolis and found that he was replacing one form of subsistence living with another. In addition, he found himself cut off from the traditional patterns that gave his life a sense of rhythm and stability in Mississippi. Disconnected from established family and community relations, he found his life being influenced by the pull of the streets and the allure of their temporary pleasures. As he became involved in gambling, prostitution-related activities, running around, drinking, and hustling, Mr. Green had discovered a new lifestyle, as had many black men who migrated to American cities during the 1950s and 1960s. It is fair to say that, in part, he lived much of his life as a "poster boy" for moral turpitude and personal irresponsibility, the kind of life that would feed the stereotypical judgments made by so many about the inner-city black man.

However, in getting to know J. W. during his time of serious illness, I saw a different side of him and was able to understand how many of his actions were traceable to the terrible hardness of his life. Although the impact of extreme poverty that was his "birthright" can never be precisely defined or measured, there is no doubt that it held sway over his view of the world and his actions in it. To get to know J. W. was to see poverty deeply rooted in him, impressed in him by his experiences in both the rural and urban settings in which he lived, yet there was a side to him that was insightful, courageous, grateful, deeply spiritual, and concerned about others. As with Cowboy, I often imagined how his life might have turned out had he not been forced to endure the difficulties and injuries of economic deprivation. In fact, his strength and regard for others was apparent when I first met him. In conversation with family and friends, he offered instructions on coping with illness:

> I got cancer. Yeah. I got it. Yeah. You're sure? [someone inter-
> rupted]. They said we are sure as sure can be, because we've
> tested it. They said we can treat cancer, but we can't promise we
> are going to kill it. There is no cure for it.

He continued:

> Whatever I got is mine. Doesn't belong to no one else. I can live
> with this. I ain't gonna try to die. I am going to try to live with this.

Then he made eye contact directly:

> You all do what you have to do. This doesn't scare me at all. You
> live as long as you can. I got to live with this, you see. This is mine.
> Y'all go about your business like you would. If anything happens
> to me, if I don't feel good, I'll let you know. Don't want you all to
> worry about me.

J. W. was waging at least two battles. The obvious one was his fight against cancer. Less obvious, but of equally compelling importance, was his struggle to pre-
serve independence and dignity. In some ways this was the more important one for
him to win. As he said on many occasions, dying was not his primary worry.
Rather, he was concerned that in physical decline he would become an ordeal for
others, burdening them with caretaking responsibilities while leaving him feeling
ashamed and humiliated in forced dependency.

> I don't think about dying, nothing like that. I am going to die any-
> way. I might as well make the best of my life while I got it. The only
> thing that I've thought about is that I don't want to be a burden on
> my people. I am not going to be that. I don't want to be nursed or
> cleaned and all washed up, or something like that, or some other
> kind of handicap. This is the only thing I wouldn't want to get into.

In his own way, without fanfare or noticeable effort, J. W. was preparing for death, not
looking forward to it, certainly, but nonetheless accepting it as a natural part of his life.

In order to give himself "every chance to live," J. W. eagerly and hopefully
agreed to be treated aggressively for his cancer. Like so many inner-city poor, he
understood very little about the disease, the treatment, or the options available to
him. He placed himself in the care of his doctors in the oncology clinic, doctors
whose names he did not know or seemingly even care to know. For the most part,
he simply trusted both their intentions and skill, thereby becoming cooperative and
compliant in his care. His lack of understanding, in part rooted in poor communication with his doctors, did become a persistent source of frustration, however, and
it was one about which he regularly complained:

I ain't sure what's happening. That's right. I would like to know
more about my condition. I would like to know more. I want them
to tell me if this cancer may last me the rest of my life. How long
or short it is, I don't know. What are they going to do to my body,
or what not, I don't know that either.

J. W. knew he had prostate cancer. He also knew it had spread to the bone. He understood nothing about the extent of its spread or its prognosis. He knew little, if
anything, about the course of treatment he was on. He responded poorly to his earlier treatment, and his doctors, fearing that he would be dead in less than a year,
became interested in enrolling him in a protocol whereby he would receive experimental chemotherapy. They talked briefly with him about this option and gave him
all the information along with enrollment forms to take home and study. His knowledge about the purpose and goals of this protocol was scant. He understood only
that if he signed up for it, he would "have to go through this long-term program
they have out there." Despite the fact that on the first page of the protocol it was
stated that he was being invited to participate in the study because he had an "abnor-
mal and serious form of cancer for which there is no standard treatment available,"
he did not understand the gravity of his situation or the extent of his disease. In fact,
even after he completed his standard course of treatment, he believed that he was
still being actively treated for his cancer. This went on for months until someone in
the radiation clinic told him, "You ain't on nothing for your cancer now. It's pain,
blood pressure, and water pills." Under the impression that he was still being treated
for his cancer, this news left him feeling more confused than ever.

I just want to know. I want to know just about what they know.
They ain't showed me no X-rays, and the first team of doctors, I
forget his name now, left and went to another state or somewhere
like that. He was gonna show me my X-rays and stuff like that because I want X-rays and stuff like that. They would be trying to explain what they saw in 'em, you know? Well, he left. And they, the
two other doctors down there now and they ain't told me nothing!
They ain't told me nothing!

J. W. would often say that his cancer felt "low, real low." "I don't think it's advanced any," he would go on to say repeatedly over a period of months. These
months were characterized by physical decline, making his self-assessment contradictory to observable physical reality, and despite this belief that the cancer was
"still low," he suffered increasing pain.

It came right across the backbone, right in here. Then it came
right across the neck and came down to the shoulder area, right
in here . . . and, it seems to be getting worse. I don't get to sleep
until about three or four o'clock in the morning. It's also very un-

comfortable because I have hard sweats, you know. I break out in
sweats about every four or five hours.

Additionally, his legs were becoming steadily weaker, and he was dizzy most of the
time. He had difficulty walking, and even in the house he had to use a cane to get
around. His declining physical condition and the increasing pain threatened his denial.
In this frame of mind, in which his thoughts were drifting back and forth from
worry to denial, he would again complain, "They are not telling me the whole
story." When asked how much he wanted to know, he quickly responded, "Tell me
the whole story."

"The whole story Mr. Green?"

"The whole story. That's right."

"For real?"

"Yep. For real. Dying ain't wrong. When it comes down to living and dying, you
need to prepare yourself for anything, especially when you get to a certain age."

Despite the idealistic scenarios described by providers in Chapter 3, it is no secret
that many physicians, including oncologists, have difficulty entering into open, candid
conversations about the end of life. Taking refuge in clinical details, they often
leave patients feeling they have not been told everything and speculating about
their condition. I will go on record here and state that from the point of view of
patients, this is unfair. It not only elicits concern about "what they are not telling
me," it inhibits the ability of patients and families to prepare for death and
make timely choices

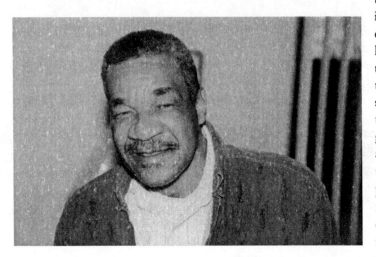

A mischievous smile graces his face as J. W. talks about girlfriends and
life on the streets.

that will improve quality of life. In order to do well by their patients, especially when
they are so disarmed and rendered vulnerable by serious disease, doctors need to become competent in skills that extend beyond the clinical. Patients especially need to be
assured that their physicians will not abandon them during this difficult time. They also
need honesty tempered with patient-centered empathy. If patients begin to sense that

their doctors are not telling them everything, the typical result is heightened frustration, worry, and anger. When this occurs, trust, which is critical in the doctor–patient relationship, is supplanted by suspicion and doubt. This is precisely what happened to J. W. because inadequate communication created extensive cogitation and agitation, which left him feeling angry with his doctors.

In addition to experiencing pain, feeling frustrated, and wondering about the future, J. W. was grieving the loss of physical vitality. He bemoaned his weakness, attributing it to age rather than cancer: "The only thing I really miss about my life is my age. My muscles aren't hard no more; I don't have the strength I used to. I feel like I got it, but it ain't there." He went on to talk about his sexual yearnings with the same sense of loss, complaining that there was no way for him to relieve or satisfy his urges. "We are all going to miss these things I guess, but they was really important to me most of the time." Struggling to hold on to life as he knew it, J. W. still had a "stable of girlfriends," as he called it:

> I got so many girlfriends. They call me all the time, but I can't really do anything. I let them know that. I don't hide anything from them. I tell them all of the time that I can't have sex with them.

He went on, without embarrassment, to describe how he liked to get naked, kiss, and fool around.

> Yep, I go to bed with them, and it tickles me. I like the reaction they have. "What's wrong with you?" I told you what's wrong with me. It's not happening here, baby. I then make them feel they should leave me alone and move on. They generally answer, "No, I enjoy being with you. I enjoy being with you all of the time."

The women that J. W. saw were those he knew from running the streets. They were his friends, but they were also hustlers. They hustled him for gifts and money. "I take care of them and they take care of me. They say, 'We'll be with you as long as you treat us nice and we'll treat you nice.' So, yeah, I got girlfriends young and old." He told me unashamedly that "being nice" to them was usually defined as a $20 payment. In some ways, despite feeling loss over his inability to function sexually, J. W. was able to maintain some sense of himself as a sexual person, and it should also be noted that he did so in a way consistent with his lifestyle as a street hustler.

In the middle of all this physical, medical, and personal chaos, J. W. became reflective about dying. Genuinely unafraid of death, he would discuss his view of dying without anxiety or worry:

> God is heaven. That's right. God lives within us. When we die and this body is dead, God is out of my body. He is no longer with me because I go back to the beginning. I go back to where I come

from—the earth. Yep, that's where your body is going to go—back
to the earth.

When asked if the thought of returning to the earth and decomposing in a grave
bothered him, he replied,

> Nope. You decay right there. But there is no pain. You are at
> peace. This is what death is all about. Death brings peace and no
> pain to the body.

He continued,

> That's right, no pain. Once you are dead, death has to do its thing.
> You see, death ain't with me now. But when death comes at me, I
> am dead. I am going to be dead. You see I understand that. We all
> got death. When my time comes on when death comes into my
> body and takes my soul away, it's going to leave my body there for
> you to see and process and what not.

In this conversation J. W. spoke of death almost as a friend. The simplicity of
this description along with his sense of acceptance may have mirrored the natural
rhythm of life and death in the agrarian setting of his youth. In addition, his emotional composure in the shadow of death was rooted in his faith in God. He believed that God would take care of him after death and that his soul would become
part of God and His love. In his conversations about death, he would often refer to
death's capacity for healing, even calling it once a "gift from God." In this framework J. W. perceived death directly through his experiences of living in poverty,
thereby viewing death as a form of relief from earthly struggles,

> Sure, God will take care of me after I die. Because you don't need
> no keep. You don't need no keep. You don't have to eat. You don't
> have to sleep. You don't have no pain. You are well taken care of
> after death.

J. W. anticipated that death would bring comfort, a comfort, however, that was
linked intimately to the sufferings that poverty inflicts on both body and person
throughout life. Although most affluent Americans fear death because it separates
them from the pleasures and possessions in their lives, the poor often view death as
a release from the misery of poverty. A relationship between economic privilege
and mortality is again suggested here. Affluent people, who have so much to lose,
are terrified of death because it threatens to strip away that which they worked to
amass and around which they organized their lives. On the other hand, death takes

away the indignity and sting of poverty, bringing a longed-for sense of peace and calm to those who are poor. Thus, for the more affluent, dying may often be cruel and punishing, while the poor may see it as a salve that heals.

The strength and insight of J. W. is notable in his reflections on dying. It was especially during these serious conversations that I came to believe that surely a man who exhibited such strength in the midst of bodily deterioration would have been capable of dealing with full and open disclosure from his oncologists. He wanted it, suffered because it was not forthcoming, and deserved to have had it.

As I got to know J. W. better on my frequent visits to his home, I became a sort of adopted member of his family. I did not know it at first, but quite early in our relationship he would tell others about this "great friend from the medical center," who came to visit and listen to him. "Just to talk?" they would inquire, and he would respond "Yep!" Our relationship became important to him, perhaps because he lived with deep fears of abandonment. As he noted:

J. W.: *I think about God all the time. I say my prayers everyday.*

DAVID: *What kind of prayers do you say?*

J. W.: *I thank God for you taking time to come out and sit down and talk with me.*

DAVID: *You thank God for me coming out.*

J. W.: *I thank God for you coming out.*

DAVID: *Why do you do that?*

J. W.: *I don't know. I thought about you when I was down in Mississippi. When I was down there I told my sisters and nieces that I got a guy that comes out to my house to interview me and talk about my problems, just like he was my brother or sister. And I thought about you a whole lot of time since I been back in. William, I asked him a couple of times, has the doctor called recently? [Although he knew that I am an educator and Ph. D., J. W. referred to me as "Doc".] We've got to have him come back to our home. He said, "No, he ain't called." And then when time goes away, "Well, he called the other day. He wants to set up an appointment." You called here last weekend. Yeah, we talked about you all the time.*

DAVID: *That's nice to hear.*

J. W.: *We sure do. Because you come out and sit down and talk with us. You come out all the time and you been in this home ever since. Even way down South. They ask, "He come out to your house?" I say, "Yeah, he come out here. He comes out here and sits down and talks to me." They ask, "What you all talk about?" "We talk about everything—dying, getting older, getting handicapped, or whatnot." You see, a lot of my thoughts and ideas about living, I kept them to myself most of the time. And when you ask me questions like that, I can freely express it. Because most folk doesn't want you to express your sickness to them.*

There is deep wisdom in these simple words. Unwittingly, J. W. was describing the value of *mindful presence* and *conscious listening* in relieving suffering. Traditionally in American culture, communal support saw the dying person and loved ones into and through death. In this context, extended family connections and community presence served to ease the burden of dying and grieving. Unfortunately, today many people endure the last months of life in significant isolation and loneliness. J. W.'s words are an important reminder that consistent caring presence is an essential element of relieving suffering and improving the quality of life's end. If Americans are ever going to become serious about reshaping the end of life, the problem of the detachment and exile of the dying will have to be prominent in that effort. This is nowhere more the case than for the inner-city poor, who are particularly detached and abandoned in a culture of materialism and individualism.

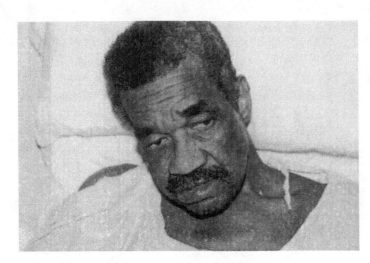

Living in the nursing home, J. W. is haunted by feelings of loneliness and isolation.

Despite genuine optimism of spirit, J. W.'s body was in a state of rapid decline. Becoming increasingly incapable of self-care, he found himself increasingly isolated. He did not have family who were willing and able to take care of him. Thus, in consultation with his doctors, the decision was made to move him to Deerfield village. Having lived with his nephew and his wife, William and Georgia, in a familiar and comfortable setting for the previous two years, the move was unsettling. For several reasons, including a fear of hospitals and doctors, William did not come to visit him in the nursing home. This separation from his nephew left J. W. feeling frightened and lonely. Additionally, his sons, to whom he had not been the best of fathers, were nowhere to be found. The result was that J. W. experienced a crushing feeling of isolation during his first days in the nursing home.

In the chaos and loneliness of settling into the nursing home, another nephew came to visit. Frank, a fifty-year-old man, cared very much about his uncle. Seeing his distress and listening to him complain about being neglected and rejected, Frank promised J. W. that he would see him through till the end. J. W., visibly nervous about being alone, began to cling to Frank desperately. For the first few nights, Frank was so worried about "Unc," as he called him, that he kept a twenty-four-hour-a-day vigil over J. W. and slept in a chair next to his bed.

Frantic from fears of abandonment, J. W. seized Frank's presence with lockjaw intensity. Whenever Frank would leave his side, even if it were to go out to eat or walk home to take a shower, a crisis erupted. J. W. faulted Frank whenever he went away, literally assailing him with accusations of abandonment. Frank responded to these outbursts with reassurances, but it was three months before J. W. began to calm down, finally believing that his nephew was going to stay with him for the duration. J. W.'s fear of abandonment was so urgent that Frank maintained his twenty-four-hours-a-day, seven-days-a-week vigil around "Unc's" bedside for six weeks. Staff at the nursing home worried about Frank burning out, and many people talked to him about his own stress and strain. Slowly, Frank began to realize he could not maintain this schedule indefinitely. He decided he should leave the nursing home after J. W. went to sleep so he could spend the night at home. After several difficult conversations with "Unc," Frank was "granted permission" to go home to sleep. True to his word, Frank faithfully returned to J. W.'s bedside every single morning until the day he died.

The six months spent in the nursing home were an enigmatic time for J. W. Frank's dedicated support gave him enormous comfort.

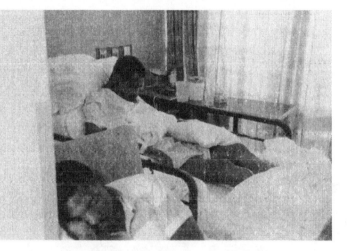

Frank maintains his twenty-four-hour presence at the bedside.

On the other hand, inadequate bedside care created anger and resulted in horrendous bedsores. He was not turned on a regular basis, and as a result his bottom became infected with painful sores that looked and smelled terrible. He was grateful when people dropped by, and he spent a lot of time fearing loneliness. His body was failing quickly, and he was becoming quadriplegic as the cancer spread up his spine. Nonetheless, he remained upbeat and cheerful most of the time.

One Wednesday afternoon we were having a candid discussion about his physical decline. Remarkably and without bitterness, J. W. relayed with confidence that "a halo of glory" was coming his way. He believed that his "disease was how I get to Jesus" and that all of his physical tribulations were part of Jesus "coming my way." We talked in detail about what it was like to lie in bed in the nursing home as a quadriplegic, and I asked him how he was coping.

"What you mean?" he queried.

"Well, Mr. Green, the things you used to do you can't do anymore. Fishing, which you love so much. Other things, like pouring a glass of water or scratching your nose. These are things you can no longer do. In light of all this, how are you feeling?"

Without hesitation, he replied, "Joy."

"Excuse me," I said, quite sure that my ears had betrayed me. "Could you say that again, please?"

Mr. Green spoke again easily and with peace of mind, "Joy is reigning/raining."

To this day I am unsure whether he meant that joy is raining, as if it might rain joy from heaven, if he meant joy is reigning, as if it were his predominant emotional state, or if the reigning God was joy. It does not matter because the result was the same. In the midst of physical suffering J. W. was able to feel serenity and jubilation because of his deep faith. During this conversation and many others he broke into spontaneous song and prayer in praise of God.

So often in our culture in which interactions with the dying are rushed and hurried, we miss the opportunity to witness the enormous bravery that lies beyond the visage of physical decline. As if he knew I was struggling to understand how he could feel joy in the face of such bodily deterioration and loss, he said later that day as I was leaving his room,

Don't worry about me. I can deal with this.

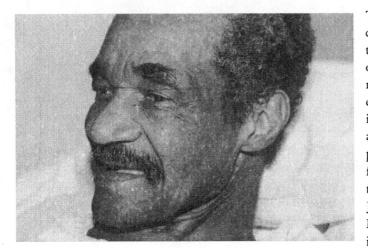

"A halo of glory is coming."

Theologians and sociologists have written about the concept of theodicy, whereby religion offers unique comfort and meaning in sickness and death, a comfort and sense of purpose that cannot be found in secular systems of meaning. J. W., like Annie Dickens, truly embodied theodicy in action.

J. W. also found comfort in simple everyday things. For example, getting to eat breakfast was a reason for celebration. "You know, I had breakfast today, and not everybody could say he had breakfast." On another occasion I brought him flowers. Upon waking and realizing that they were for him, he started to cry. He wanted to know if they were real, and he wanted to touch them. Unable to move his arm or fingers, it was necessary to lift his hand and stroke his fingers over the top of the flowers. As he first touched the flowers, he said, "Soft, like the morning dew." Continuing to touch them, he spoke about how more joy was coming to his life and said, "Thank you, thank you." Tears still flowed as the vase was put on the tray next to his bed, and after a few minutes he asked if he could touch them again.

These expressions of joy and celebration coexisted with strain and tension, and his optimism and strength were being tested daily. His pain was "getting worse," and family conflict periodically surfaced. For example, one day walking down the hallway to see J. W., Frank came running toward me crying out that "All hell is breaking loose in there!" J. W.'s nephew, William, had come to visit, and they were in a heated argument about some money that had disappeared from J. W.'s checking account. William had access to the account. J. W. suspected that he stole money, and Frank was convinced of it. Despite the probing questions being asked, however, the matter was never resolved. In fact, for the most, part J. W. never really pressed the issue. To the contrary, he sought reconciliation, hoping not to further alienate his nephew. Frank, on the other hand, was irate. He felt that William, by virtue of his infrequent visits, was not doing right by "Unc."

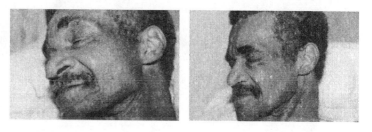

The comfort of faith and prayer.

"And now this shit happens," he complained. Tension between the two of them was intense and remained so until J. W. died. They kept their feud private, however, out of respect for J. W., who told them in no uncertain terms to "Cut it out."

In another instance J. W. was hoping to leave the nursing home and find a place to live with Frank. They were counseled against the move because his doctor and nurse felt Frank could not manage caring for "Unc" on his own. J. W. proposed that one of his sons, scheduled to be released from jail in about a month, come live with the two of them to help Frank. Frank rejected the idea because he wanted nothing to do with his cousin. That only made J. W. more insistent, and a battle between them erupted. Throughout the course of their conflict, J. W. remained visibly angry with Frank. Frank remained steadfast in his commitment to take care of his uncle but voiced strong opposition to J. W.'s plan. Frank was indignant about the idea because he felt the son's "criminal nature" would not be a good influence in either of their lives. All J. W. would say to Frank was that "This is my business, not yours." Rancor and acrimony could clearly be heard in his voice. Frank never said this in front of J. W., but he was convinced that the plan was part of an attempt by his uncle to make up for a lifetime of neglect of his children. Once again, the conflict was never resolved. Rather, it faded away because the son wanted no part of living with either of them. He was released from jail, and until the day he died J. W. never knew where he was living or how he was doing.

On another occasion, another son who had never before visited was found pilfering through J. W.'s closet in the nursing home looking for money. This took place early in September, around the time that J. W. normally received his checks. Frank caught him in the act and informed him, "There is no money here for you, so stay away." A complaint was filed with the nursing home administrator, and the son was barred from coming back. On another occasion one of J. W.'s "girlfriends" was found in bed with him. This created conflict between "Unc" and Frank because J. W. wanted her companionship, while Frank insisted that, "We have to create a new standard for your behavior." The woman, like the son, was told "There is no money for you here" and sent away. J. W., longing for the companionship of a woman, interrupted. "But that doesn't mean you can't come and see me." The woman responded as she was leaving the room, "I'll be back tomorrow." Not surprisingly, J. W. never saw her again.

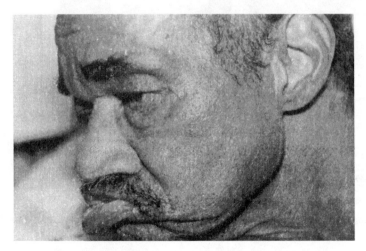

J. W. expresses dissatisfaction with the care he is receiving.

Having become both a prisoner of his body and the nursing home, J. W. began to complain about the care he was receiving. His bedsores were getting worse and becoming infected. During a brief conversation to introduce the concept of hospice, the nurse in charge of his care said to him, "Well, it all depends on how you want to go down." The insensitivity of her remark was not lost on either J. W. or Frank. In response he said, "Well, you know the attitude I am getting." He was referring to his perception that the nurses were impatient with him and often rushed him to take his medicine. Difficulty in swallowing made administering medicine a time-consuming process. Sometimes the understaffed and overworked nurses and nursing assistants, in their efforts to be quick and efficient in their work, did become irritated with him. He complained about their "disapproving frowns" and the way they "rolled their eyes," yet, like so many inner-city poor, he never complained to anyone in authority about his care. Instead, he internalized his feelings, although sometimes he expressed his dissatisfaction aloud in our conversations.

> **Well, you know, Doc. It's all about money. They've got it and I don't. I'm unimportant to them, because they do have it.**

After six months of living in the nursing home, time was running out. During the last month of his life, J. W. complained less and less about the indignities of the care he received. He seemed to have his attention on other matters, such as "going home!" For J. W. "going home" meant that he would be going to join his Lord. He craved prayer during this time. Unfortunately, sources of religious support in the nursing home were scarce. He saw his own pastor only once while at Deerfield, although they spoke occasionally on the phone. Unfortunately, despite being enrolled in hospice during the final month, a relationship with a hospice chaplain never materialized. Nevertheless, J. W. remained steadfast in his faith, praying and smiling throughout his ordeal because he felt blessed and firm in his conviction that a great reward lay ahead.

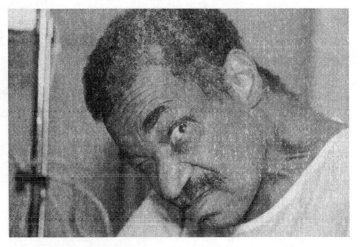

Words of wisdom and insight flow from this impoverished African American from the "other side of the tracks."

As death approached the thing he craved most, other than spiritual comfort, was human contact. Unable to move any part of his body at all, he yearned to be touched. The feel of death was apparent throughout his body, one that had been savaged by disease. Even so, despite his physical deterioration, his spirit remained strong and vital, and he longed for connectedness with others. Once when I hugged him good-bye, he started to cry. Trying to calm him, Frank immediately reached out and offered comfort, saying "It's okay, Unc. It's okay. It's okay." J. W. responded,

> **No. It feels good. It just feels so good to be hugged. I like that. It just feels so good.**

A mutual relationship had been established in our time together, for which I was grateful. He had taught me so much about a world of which I had known little and demonstrated an insuperable resilience that had its roots in the agrarian poverty of his youth. Knowing that the end of his life was rapidly approaching, I asked J. W. what message he would like to send others.

DAVID: *As I tell your story to other people, what is the one thing you want them to know?*

J. W.: *I want people to know how to love their neighbors, and love their brothers and their sisters. Tell them that we are imperfect and are going to make mistakes and hurt each other, but to keep on loving.*

DAVID: *That's the one thing you want people to understand about life?*

J. W.: *Just tell them—good morning. It's another day. I get to love you again today.*

Sage words, indeed, and spoken by a man dying in a nursing home who grew up as a tenant farmer in Mississippi. These words were shaped, perhaps, by his inability to enact them in his own life. Nevertheless, they are compelling advice from a disempowered, uneducated man who lived his life on the economic, cultural, and social margins of American society. So insightful were these words that, once again, I am forced to wonder what his life would have been like had he not had to endure the hardships and injuries of poverty in both its rural and urban configurations.

Strength in Poverty: Joe Noble

> Saying good-bye is the hard part; that is the only hard part; it's not dying.
>
> —Joe Noble

Tears were streaming down his cheeks as Joe Noble spoke of his father. "He was a great man. I worshipped him," he said from his hospital bed. "I always have worshipped him. He sacrificed so much. He gave up his own necessities so he could support us. He never said 'I love you,' but I never doubted his love and affection."

Big Sam, as Joe's father was called, was born in Kiev, Russia, at the turn of the twentieth century. A strong, strapping man, he immigrated to the United States at the age of sixteen, primarily to escape an arranged marriage and to seek a better life. He came alone, not knowing anyone in America who could offer a reassuring welcome. Just after being processed at Ellis Island, he heard a man speaking in various languages. "Who wants to work? Does anyone want to work?" As Joe relays the story, his father "went to the voice" and said he wanted to work. The fact that Big Sam was illiterate did not matter, especially after this prospective employer saw his impressive physical stature. Along with some other immigrants, he was invited to a local pub in lower Manhattan, where he was provided with pitchers of beer and ham sandwiches. Once again, he was questioned, "Do you sincerely want to work? Do you want to work hard?" Assuring the stranger that he did, Big Sam boarded a train to Canada, where he worked for several years in a logging camp. "He was a slave there," his dying son said years later with anger and bitterness in his voice. "He would sleep outside under the horses when the weather was bad, with the manure and them urinating on him. It was real bad in the winter. Winters were so cold that it took years after leaving the camp until he was able to feel warm again." Although they suffered in the cold during the harsh winters in the woods of Canada, food was plentiful. "They would always eat good," Joe reported. Nonetheless, "He would cry himself to sleep every night. He wished he was dead. Wished he had never been born, wondering what he got himself into, and wishing he had never left Russia."

One of the projects that Big Sam worked on was the Rainbow Bridge at Niagara Falls. He was involved in cutting timber and helping in the construction of the bridge, which was largely constructed of wood. While working on this project, a "little carnival" that consisted of a Ferris wheel, carousel, and several amusement booths set up camp near the workers. "My father hung around them a lot, enjoying treats such as candy. He had no family so he used to spend most of his money on tobacco and alcohol." Big Sam became a regular at the carnival, and the man who ran it had occasion to see how hard Sam worked for the lumber company. Before it left to set up operations elsewhere, Big Sam was offered a job with the carnival, which he quickly accepted. His employment with the traveling carnival enabled him to enter the United States, and he wound up in Ohio near Akron. While still working for the carnival, again "almost as a slave," he met a fellow immigrant who had lived in a neighboring village in Russia. This person informed him of a job opportunity in a local rubber factory that paid better wages than Big Sam had ever hoped to earn. When he worked "two feet in front of furnaces that burned at 1,200°F, it felt good. I didn't even sweat for two years," his father would often joke, remembering how cold his winter nights as a lumberjack had been. "This was a good job, and he made some decent money for a change," his son said, choking back tears and taking bittersweet comfort in knowing that at least for a brief period his father's struggles were eased.

Big Sam, being alone in a strange land, looked to his fellow immigrant as both a brother and father. He identified closely with the man and saw him as a mentor. Joe, on the other hand, has different memories of the man whom he bitterly described as a "bastard." "I hated him, could have killed him because all the time I knew him he did nothing but mistreat, make fun of, and belittle my father because he was illiterate. He showed him no respect at all."

This man, who always remained a giant in Big Sam's eyes, had decided that there was prestige and money to be made in the coal mines, so he convinced Sam to quit the rubber factory, relocate to western Pennsylvania, and go to work in the mines. "My father became a slave again," Joe painfully noted. For all the years he worked there, "He was able to reach $4,000 annual salary only two times, and that was because of all the overtime he put in. He supported his wife, five kids, and his wife's mother on that income until he was retired by the mine in 1958 at the age of sixty-five."

"I loved my father," Joe would often say. "I miss him so. He did everything he possibly could do for me. Going to work hungry so we could eat. I owe him every-thing. I can't ever repay him." Despite growing up poor, with the legacy of poverty continuing to be a source of struggle in his adult life and for his three children, he never faltered in his love of his father. Without any trace of bit-terness, he commented, "Yeah, I've struggled fi-nancially all my life. Yeah, we experienced hardships because of my back-ground. Adele came from a poor family, too, you know. And thing's got worse while I was disabled for a lot of years."

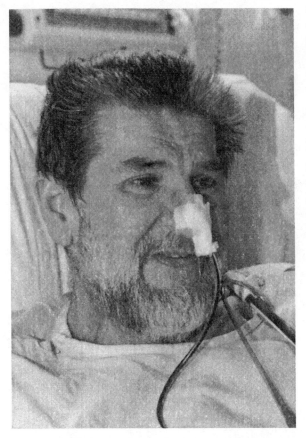

"Life is so precious. It is just so hard to give it all up. To never see the pear trees again. To know I'll never experience another Christmas. Not to be able to fish again. But most of all, it is so painful to have to say goodbye to Adele and the kids. It would all be okay if I could put them in my pocket and take them with me," remarked Mr. Noble.

He had been working as a respiratory therapist for thirteen years until he had a work-related acci-dent. "One day I was run-ning to a cardiac arrest because I was part of the team. I stepped off the ele-vator, not looking out for my own safety, and slipped and fell," Joe recalled. He injured his back so severely that he was on worker's compensation for two years. After that he lost his disability and struggled to find employment. Unsuc-cessful in attempting to re-turn to respiratory therapy, he tried selling insurance for a while. His back injury persisted and limited his capac-ity for work, so he bounced from one part-time job to another. All the while the fam-ily had to survive his periods of unemployment solely on Adele's income. She worked as a nursing assistant and made about $6 to $7 an hour.

As a matter of fact, poverty was a condition that Joe accepted as the simple real-ity of the only life he ever knew:

Our children did without, and thank God we lived thrifty. We both had had poverty in our youth. We never experienced the trappings of high society. We just wanted a comfortable life. Shelter, pay the bills, enjoying the simple things in life, you know, nature, going fishing. . . . Our children grew up as we did. We had no status or prestige. We felt discriminated against, but we never discriminated. We were the only family who ever got along with the blacks. In fact, they loved my father. When he died, there was the largest black attendance at that funeral home.

It would seem that in finding ways to cope with all the negative elements of poverty, Joe Noble had learned some important lessons in life, lessons that provided moral grounding along with the ability to cope with the tribulations of dying.

Joe's cancer was particularly insidious. "The cancer is like an octopus," that was particularly interested in "invading the intestine, bowel, and stomach," he noted. "It is very aggressive and fast growing. It has increased in size thirty percent, and the chemo has had no effect. There is no possibility of surgery as the surgery is so intricate, having to deal with all the blood vessels and all. The surgeons told me it is impossible to go in . . . and that there would be zero survival. They are talking weeks; time is real precious now." In fact, time was so precious that he did not have time for fear or anger. "No, I'm not afraid. My mental attitude is strong. I've been through dress rehearsals for death before. I've been within hours of death when they did the emergency ostomy, and I survived that. Then, when I had the abscess I was supposed to die. Prior to that I had a massive blood clot and was not expected to survive. Much prior to that was the cellutitis, taking me back three years. I was within minutes of amputation just to save my life. Throughout all of that there was no fear, and there is none now."

As I got to know Joe better, he, like Annie, took great pride in becoming my teacher. He fashioned himself a "Morrie from the other side of the tracks," referring to the book *Tuesdays with Morrie*. An undergraduate student in my death and dying class was spending ten hours a week with the Noble family as part of an internship in palliative care and gave Joe the book. "There is no shame in dying and no dishonor in death. Leaving loved ones behind, that is the only dishonor in dying," he instructed. Tears flowed from his eyes, and he struggled to find the words. "I don't know which is worse, choked up emotions or dehydrations," he said with an affected smile.

I hate it. I just hate it. Dying takes me away from everything here that is precious. Everything that we know down here. It's the farewell that is the bitch. It sucks. I love the world. I love the people I am going to leave behind. [He was sobbing almost inconsolably at this point.] Adele, the children, that's the hard part. If I could take them in my hand [He opened his palm and clenched his fingers as if they were there and he were clenching onto them.] put them in my pocket and take them with me, then I'd be ready to go. It's just so ridiculous, having to leave.

When asked how he was able to control his anger and not feel bitter at such a difficult time, he stated that he needed to stay focused on positive things so he could enjoy every minute with his family. "It's all so precious, and so many people take it for granted," he declared.

> Sure I'm angry, but I just don't want it to overwhelm me. It's just a waste of positive time. So, rage and anger is just a waste of positive energy; futile, it doesn't accomplish anything. But, I also look at what I've had; I've had fifty-two years. I've had Adele for thirty-two years, and my family for twenty-nine years. So, see, I've had so much. I'd like a thousand years or eternity, but I've got no regret. I have had her companionship; relationships are what it is all about.

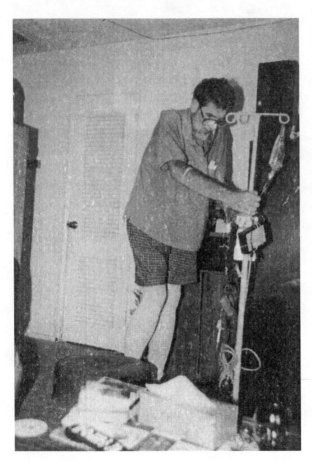

Disease destroyed Joe's body but never conquered his love of life.

The words were dramatically similar to Morrie's. Maybe Joe was right in thinking that he was "Morrie from the other side of the tracks!" He continued.

> Saying good-bye is hard. That is the only hard part. It is not dying. I know they don't want me to go, either. In fact, my experience is nothing compared to theirs. They are facing the hard part. Adele, sometimes we sit and think about it, and it all seems so impossible. As hard as it all seems, we look back without regret. Sometimes when we would get lost in the material stuff, and be depressed over what we didn't have, we would always get back to basics—human basics

and our family. If I have one regret, I regret not showing love—expressing it. I wasn't as verbal as I should have been. I hate myself now for not saying I love you more often. I got that from my father, you know? But, during the past two years, boy, have I overcompensated. . . . Yes. I'm a better person now because of being sick. One-hundred percent a better husband, father, and person.

It is important to remember that Joe lived everyday in discomfort and pain. He had had no solid food for nine months. He was receiving nutrition intravenously by a process called total parenteral alimentation. For the past three years he had found himself in and out of the hospital. Given the extent of the disease, he was correct in stating that his strength, both mental and physical, was the reason he had survived so long. There were times, however, when that was a mixed blessing. For example, one Friday afternoon he was rushed to the emergency room (ER) in exquisite pain. The slightest movement brought agony, and he was in so much discomfort that he almost could not tolerate the simple X-rays that had been ordered. The first nurse who at-

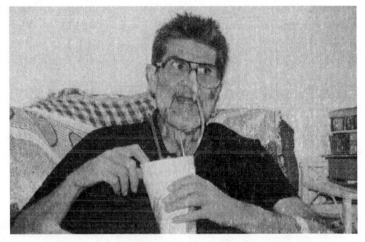

Unable to eat any food, Joe would pour a little root beer over ice chips and then dump the soda out. "Just to give it a little flavor," he would say.

tended him compassionately instructed, "If this morphine doesn't help in ten to fifteen minutes, you let us know. We have plenty more, and there is no need for you to suffer."

Writhing in his bed in the observation unit, Joe struggled to gain mental focus and control of the pain, but it did not work. About twenty minutes later Adele went to the nurses' station to find his nurse. Unfortunately, she had been sent to the urgent visit center next door to finish her shift and was no longer working on Joe's case. When Adele told the replacement nurse that he needed more medicine, she snapped, "He just had some!"

"He's in so much pain, he needs more," Adele replied.

The nurse responded begrudgingly, "I'll have to check with the doctor." When Adele came back to him, Joe's body was convulsed in pain. He kept saying over and over, "If only I weren't so strong, this would be over by now. It would be over." A tear made its way down his left cheek. Adele wiped his forehead, telling him she loved him and that it would be okay. Two hours and two additional injections later, the pain began to subside. Joe was sent home about 9:00 PM that evening, the ER doctor having told him there was nothing that could be done except to try to help him get through the episodes of severe pain.

In the midst of all this suffering and despite the words of despair he uttered in the ER, Joe embraced life. If he said it once, he said it a hundred times: "It's so precious." When I asked if there was one particular message he would want to relay to those who would one day hear a bit of his story, he said,

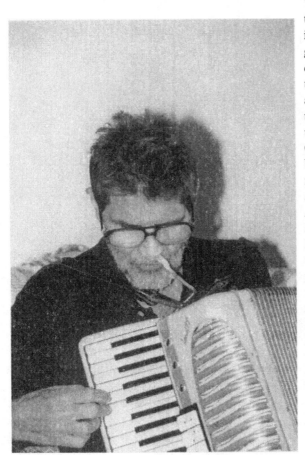

Joe's gift: A musical Popsicle.

You tell them two things: First, it is impossibly, unimaginably difficult to die. To never see the pear trees again; to know that I am not going to have another Christmas; not to be able to fish anymore; but most of all never to see Adele and the kids again. It's all too hard. You tell them that. Second, you tell them that what they do is so important. To relieve suffering and help comfort me while I am dying, I cannot imagine more important work.

Consistent with these "lessons from Joe," as I have come to call them, Mr. Noble, despite all his suffering, treasured life and those he loved. He yearned for life and to experience it in connection with others. Sometimes he would organize an entire week around an hour's fishing outing. Invariably, it would take a toll on his body, worsening his pain and other symptoms, but it was "worth the price" for him to remain engaged in something he enjoyed so much and something he could do with his family. On one occasion during an especially memorable home visit that Jodi and I made two weeks before his death, he shared his feelings for us.

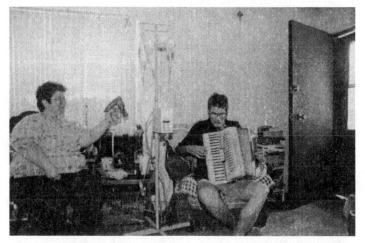

Adele joins in the celebration with bubbles, á la Lawrence Welk.

You are a part of my life. Just yourselves. Your sympathetic, humanistic self has been a part of me. Your group. You are two of the most caring human beings that I've ever met. I wished I had known you longer. I am going to miss you! I know I will continue on through you. This was planned even before we were born, that we should meet like this. I have a gift for you.

At that point Joe and Adele disappeared to another room, and when they returned she was carrying his accordion. "I haven't played it for years, but I thought I'd give it a try for your group."

Over the next thirty minutes, Joe struggled to play. The accordion

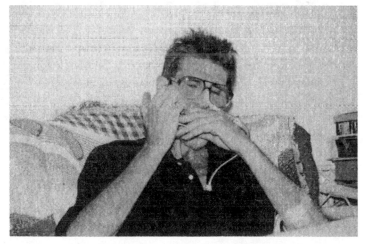

Physically unable to play the squeezebox any longer but not yet finished with his gift, Joe plays "Danny Boy" on the harmonica.

was heavy, but he was still strong enough to manage it. The biggest difficulty was feeling "the Braille," as he called the keys. His fingers were insensate from the morphine, and he struggled to find the appropriate notes. The music he made, while not technically perfect, was spine tingling and beautiful. After about a half an hour, he was unable to play the "squeeze box" any longer, but he was not yet finished giving his gift. He got out his harmonica, and we were held captive by every note he played of "Coming Round the Mountain," "Sunshine," and "Danny Boy." I have often had the opportunity to play the tape for audiences when I lecture, and they, like us, find Joe's gift to be spiritually moving and reflective of a deep and intimate bond between caring professionals from the public hospital and a dying man from "across the tracks."

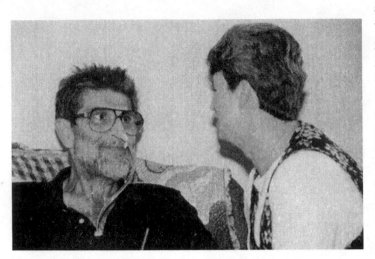

Jodi and Joe express their love.

The following poem, entitled "Popsicle" and written by Philips Cozzie, M.D., appeared recently in *Annals of Internal Medicine*. The patient written about is at the threshold of death, however his final request is one that embraces life, returning to a time when life was carefree and joyful. One last time, as the poem reveals, he wants to revel in the taste, texture, and joy of being alive:

> Remember running in cutoffs on hot hot summer afternoons
> directly across neighbor's lawns, through sprinklers, across
> curbs,
> Toward the jingling bells and the man in white hustling treats
> from the side of a truck. We were stunned into silence by the
> vast array of choices. Wahoo bars, only five cents. Who could
> afford a toasted almond bar? Nothing compared to a sloppy
> melting lime or banana twin Popsicle. Twin Popsicles, best
> separated on the edge of a table by a quick hit with the ball of
> the hand, were twice as good.
> Remember sucking the end so hard that all the juice ran up

and out, leaving only a white skeleton of a Popsicle.
We each negotiated the final nubbin of frozen ice on a stick in
individual ways. So it didn't surprise me, thirty years later, to
learn that Mr. Bowers requested, five minutes before support
was withdrawn, a Popsicle, as if reveling in the choices
remaining for him and all the dying. He ran back through
time to the squish of feet on watered grass, the luscious crush
of Popsicle on tongue.

For Joe, playing these instruments one last time for people that he had grown to
deeply care about was akin to one last taste of Popsicle. One last time he was able
to make music, laugh, and share a moment of joy. Seemingly, Joe sensed that the
end was near. Forty-eight hours from the time he played these songs, he was
bedridden. Two weeks later, his suffering finally ended as he died peacefully at
home. Adele and his children were by his side.

He was a person who was deeply grateful—for the beauty in life, for the splen-
dor of nature that soothed his soul, for Adele, for his children, for the sacrifices his
beloved father made for the sake of the family, and for the care he received at
County. In a culture of materialism in which affluence and celebrity are the dominant icons in public life, Joe and others like him are pushed to the periphery, and
their lives seemingly matter little. One more time I am reminded of King Lear and
suggest that, like the king's robes, the trappings of materialistic society are "sophisticated." But, "the thing itself," truly is the remarkable dignity and grace of the
suffering human being that was Joe Noble. Hopefully, we will all remember the lessons he wanted us to learn:

- Life is precious and should never be taken for granted.
- Dying is unimaginably difficult.
- Offering comfort to dying persons not only relieves suffering but also ennobles
  and enriches the caregiver.

Wise words, indeed, from Mr. Noble, also known as "Morrie from across the
tracks."

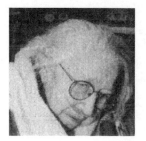

TRIUMPH AND FAITH THROUGH HARSH REALITY AND PERSONAL TRAGEDY: LUCILLE ANGEL

At the first of every dawn, I thank Him for the beginning of another day starting in my life.

—Lucille Angel

Lucille Angel was a beautiful sixty-two-year-old African-American woman who was dying of lung cancer. Like so many indigent and dying persons, Mrs. Angel rarely complained about her life. The cancer that ravaged her body left her mind intact and her spirit strong. Rather than lament her sufferings, she spent much of the time during her final months being thankful for where her life was and reflecting on what she had done in the past. "It's taken me back over my life, you know. I've thought about things that I probably should have done, and all the things I could've done better, or differently, or something like that. It's taken me back over my life."

In her contemplations and remembrances she fondly recalled her childhood in Kentucky. "We were poor—dirt poor—but we had a big family, and we had love in that house, food to eat, and a roof over our head. Nine of us. We were poor folk, but there was love in the house. I used to tell my kids I wish that they could've been raised in a loving household like I was, but they were not."

Regrettably, Mrs. Angel married a man right after leaving high school who physically abused her for nearly two decades. The consequences of that marriage still haunted her when I first met her, which was soon after she was diagnosed with cancer for the second time. Witnessed by all three of her daughters, the abuse was severe.

"I went to see doctors because I would be so beat up and everything." Once, "I stayed in bed, I could not move, I had been beaten so bad. The doctor came in to treat me and gave me a shot and asked me what happened, you know. 'Did your husband do this?' And I said, 'Of course he did,' and that was all that was said." The ideal of the old-fashioned family doctor who cares about his patients was never a reality for Mrs. Angel, especially at this point in County's history, when most of society was still living in the "dark ages" when it came to domestic violence. "They treated you and that was it. No more was said about it, until maybe you had to call them next time or else end up in the damn morgue or something."

Mrs. Angel did not pity herself because of that marriage, but she regretted the effects it had on her daughters. "I'm not making excuses for myself, but at that time, just fresh out of high school, just married from Mom and Dad's house to a husband's house, not having any kind of work skills, experience or anything. That was all I knew. And then having three children right quick. I didn't think there was any other way except to stay there and take that abuse, and that's why I blame myself. I blame myself sometimes for staying. I should've been stronger. I should've got out before I did."

In addition to physical abuse, her daughters also witnessed adultery, drug abuse, and a kind of cruel indifference from their father. The oldest daughter reminded her, "Mama, I remember the times he would pass in the summertime, with the top back on the convertible, with his girlfriends and children in the car." Mrs. Angel adds, "And he would pass right by the three of my daughters—his daughters—and not even pick them up. This has got to be hurtin' for a child."

Throughout this marriage Mrs. Angel attended church and was advised by her pastor to try not to antagonize her husband. Her husband eventually left the family and moved to Oklahoma, where he remarried.

The next chapter of Mrs. Angel's life, beginning at age forty-six, was much happier. A strong and handsome man named Mike had loved her from afar for years. He was a boxer and had been a sparring partner for the noted heavyweight boxer Archie Moore. He was a deacon in the church and had been encouraging Mrs. Angel to leave her husband for years. When her marriage to her first husband dissolved, she married Mike and once again had a loving household, as she had in childhood. She lit up as she described it. "Oh, it was the best. He was such a good person, so good and kind and understanding. He wasn't my children's natural father, but he . . . was the only father that they really knew, and they needed a father." He was also a grandfather to her children's children. "He was here long enough to see the two grandchildren, and they just loved him, too. He was just a good person, so good and kind. He was good."

During this period Mrs. Angel developed cancer in her vocal cords. She received six or seven weeks of radiation therapy, and when she finished her doctor told her he did not see any sign remaining of cancer. He told her to quit smoking, and she had not had a cigarette since.

When Lucille and Mike had been together for twelve years, Mike developed cancer. His weights sat unused in the house as his body withered. "He was a strong person, but that cancer just brought him down." Not surprisingly, Mrs. Angel cared for him at home throughout his illness and into death. "We had a hospital bed right over there for him and a wheelchair and one of those little potty things. He'd lay right there on his hospital bed and look out that window, and friends would be coming to visit him."

Mike remained emotionally uncomplaining in the face of his pain. "The doctor had prescribed morphine for him, and he wouldn't take it. I know he'd be in pain, because he would be praying. He'd be praying, 'Lord, have mercy.'" Mrs. Angel continued:

> He fought as long as he could. But then the night that he died I was sitting up with him and rubbing his hand . . . and I was talking to him, and he started asking the Lord to have mercy on him. . . . I don't know whether he was more or less tired of fighting or ready to go, but he was in so much pain, and he never would take that morphine. The night that he died I just took it and dumped it down the toilet. It hurt me so bad when I lost him, it just hurt me. I thought I'd never stop hurting. . . . I think about it now, and I almost start crying.

That sadness was followed by more distressing events. The family was beginning to return to normal activities after Mike's death, and Mrs. Angel focused her energy on planning for a big Thanksgiving meal, as she had always done. "I had done all my shopping and everything, and just a few little things I needed, so I walk down to 7-11. It was a nice day, and I strolled and took my time strolling. I picked up a few things, and was strollin' on back. Now, when I walk down that way I can see my husband's grave right from the fence, from the sidewalk. It's right there. And when I passed on down I was okay. I glanced over there, but I went on to the store and came on back. And before I quite got to his grave, I just . . . I just had a stroke. I didn't know what was happening to me. I couldn't move, and I kept dropping my purse. I wanted to come across the street down there, but you know how busy that is. Something told me, 'Don't get in that street! It's gonna be it! Cars will not stop for you.' It seemed like I was just motionless, could not move, and I kept trying to walk, thinking if I took my time maybe I could make it home. I just couldn't. I just collapsed right there."

Finally, a man stopped and offered to drive her home. He was unable to get her into his car and called an ambulance. Mrs. Angel ended up in the hospital for the Thanksgiving holidays. She said she "just felt like, 'Lord, what else can happen to me?'"

Mrs. Angel was left with deficits on her right side after her stroke. She had a great deal of pain in her right shoulder, numbness, and minimal function in her right hand. She also was having difficulty breathing. Dr. Lipton, her primary care doctor, ordered X-rays and discovered a spot on her lung. She informed Mrs. Angel that she had cancer. She could pursue surgery to remove the tumor from her lung, or she could have chemotherapy. The news was overwhelming. "I was devastated. I just couldn't believe it, you know. It was hard for me to believe, and I was very upset. I think that was one reason that I waited so long. She called me to say that I had been missing appointments, and I said, 'I don't recall missing any appointment!' I always wrote them on the calendar, but somehow or other I didn't write these on the calendar, because I guess I wasn't ready to accept it and talk to her about it."

Mrs. Angel finally met with Dr. Lipton and informed her that she did not wish to have surgery. Her decision was based on the experiences of both her husband and brother, who had undergone surgery for cancer but had died anyway. As it had been four months since her diagnosis, Mrs. Angel did not consider surgery at that

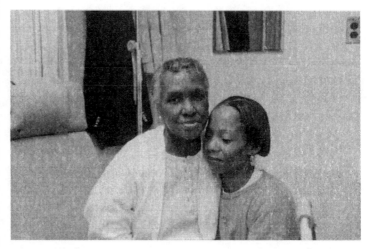

A hopeful Mrs. Angel receives chemotherapy and the love of her daughter Tawana.

time to be a viable option in any case. She found her doctor "very considerate and sympathetic. She did make it a point to let me know that there was something that could be done about it. She let me know that it's not giving up time!"

Mrs. Angel was referred to the oncology clinic, where she was taken care of by Dr. Lens. As described in Chapter 3, it was unclear when she was first diagnosed whether this was a recurrence of her earlier throat cancer or a new cancer. They began treating her with medicines that would be appropriate if it were a recurrence. She was receiving this chemotherapy as an in-patient when I first met her. She was sitting up in her hospital bed with bags of chemotherapy and intravenous fluids infusing over the course of several days. She was wearing a beautiful pink robe, and her hair was done perfectly. She invited me to sit down wherever I could find a spot. It was in this first conversation that I heard about Mike, who was clearly more on her mind than was her own cancer.

Mrs. Angel was open and gracious from the onset. She spoke of her beloved husband, his painful death, her faith in God, and her love for her family. I sat comfortably by her side, impressed with her poise and beauty while she talked lovingly about what was important in her life. Mrs. Angel liked the in-patient chemotherapy treatment because she liked her nurses and the companionship at the hospital. In fact, Mrs. Angel's favorite television show was a raucous talk show hosted by Jerry Springer, and the nurses would gather in her room to watch it with her. Once a physician came to examine her while everyone was in her room watching the show. She explained, "He asked, 'Is that Springer?' I said, 'It sure is, whatever you're getting ready to do; hurry up and do it and go out!' He just died laughing." Later, as our relationship developed and I visited her at home, she would often say, "I just love to hear from you and see you. You are welcome to call and come anytime. Just not between 10:00 AM and 11:00 AM or 4:00 PM and 5:00 PM." Thinking that perhaps this was a quiet, prayerful period during the day for her, I asked why she wanted to remain undisturbed during these particular times. She immediately responded, "Springer!" This devotion to the Springer show, seemingly so out of character for the Mrs. Angel I knew, became a source of amusement for both of us. Sometimes we would watch it together, but I was under strict orders not to disrupt her attention by talking except during commercials. To this day I cannot help but smile when I remember how this kind, gentle, and religious woman was so enthralled by a program so inconsistent with these qualities.

Although being diagnosed with cancer was a difficult and stressful experience for Mrs. Angel, perhaps she was comforted by the fact that the radiation treatment she had received ten years before had been so successful. She was hoping to be cured again in the same way. When she returned to the oncology clinic after two rounds of in-patient chemotherapy to evaluate her body's response to the medicine, she was hopeful.

She went to her appointment thinking she would find out whether she had two or four rounds of chemotherapy remaining. Instead, the oncology fellow who examined her informed her that they were changing the regimen altogether because the first medicine had had no effect on her cancer. In fact, her tumor had grown. She was so upset and surprised by this news that she cried and had trouble breathing. The fellow wondered if she needed oxygen, and Dr. Lens, her staff oncologist, went to see her. She left that appointment very angry with him. She felt he had made a grave error in her care:

> I got angry. I didn't mean to, and I did apologize to him. . . . I don't know what I said, but I know I was very angry and upset, and I probably said some things I shouldn't have said.

Although she felt ashamed of her anger, the feeling persisted.

> He was the one who started the treatment, recommended the treatment. So, who else was I to tell except him? Nine days of living in a hospital bed hooked up to all this stuff. I was angry.

When asked if she was upset because he had made a mistake or because she had had unnecessary treatments, she answered:

> Both. He's a doctor, he's a doctor. And I know they're only human, but when you go to a doctor, you need help. And that's what you expect from your doctor. . . . Don't give me a wrong diagnosis or something like that. No, the diagnosis of cancer was right, but they weren't treating it in the right place or the right manner.

Dr. Lens returned to the staff workroom after this difficult encounter and said aloud to everyone there, "I am afraid that she needs some good old-fashioned hand-holding today." Mrs. Angel also recognized that some of her anger stemmed from the fact that she had been expecting something entirely different at her appointment and had been caught off guard.

> I was under the impression that I was getting along, doing pretty good, which I was. I was upset about the fact that I went back to see him with the expectations of him telling me how many more of those treatments that I had left, either two or four more. See, I had this all made up in my mind what I wanted to know from him and I guess what I wanted to see and what I wanted to hear him say, but it wasn't like that.

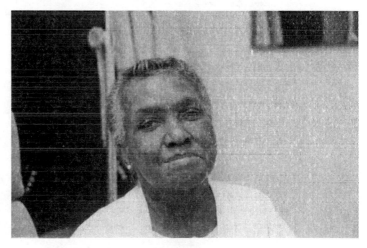

Mrs. Angel fights her anger toward her doctors and God after having received bad news in the oncology clinic.

Her main complaint from her first form of chemotherapy had been diminished appetite. The second form of chemotherapy was given to her at the oncology clinic instead of in the hospital, and it took about six hours to infuse intravenously. Several weeks later this medicine caused her to lose her hair. She had taken a shower and was combing her hair when it began to fall out in her hands. She said, "I knew it was going to happen, but it just frightened me. . . . I just started screaming and shaking all over." Her daughter Joleen and her granddaughter came into the bathroom to comfort her.

Mrs. Angel immediately felt ashamed of herself for reacting so dramatically to her hair loss.

> They make wigs every day and after I thought about it I said this is really picky. Getting upset and crying and screaming and shaking all over hair, you know what I mean? I felt real petty, real bad. . . . So many other people are losing their lives and they've lost loved ones, and for me to be so upset and emotional about some hair, I felt really bad.

For months she lived with the tension between feeling humiliated over her hair loss and feeling ashamed of her vanity. She seemed similarly disturbed by her loss of physical attractiveness and her inability to simply accept this loss as part of God's plan for her.

During this time Mrs. Angel remained unknowing and uncertain about what was happening with her disease. Her oncologist had mentioned that he might switch her medication to pill form, which Mrs. Angel assumed to mean that her second regimen was not working. "I haven't talked to him about that, but it must not be responding to the other treatments if they are getting ready to put me on a third different treatment."

Mrs. Angel, like many other patients, affirmed several times that she wished her doctor would give her more information. When I asked if she wished she knew if the treatments were working, she first answered, "Yes," but then went on. "I don't ask as many questions as I used to, and I guess by me not asking a bunch of questions, I don't get too many answers." She added, "I feel like if it was something that I really wanted to know I would ask and he would tell me the truth . . . I guess."

Although she did not press her oncologist for details about her illness, she assumed it would be fatal. She stated that she expected to die from cancer unless she got "hit by a big Mack truck." She had some hope in relation to the illness, but sometimes it was extremely hard for her to articulate what it was that she hoped for:

> I hope for a cure. I pray for a cure, but I don't. I don't know how to put it. I guess not for a cure for myself. . . . Sure I do, but I don't dwell on it. I know one day they will have a cure for cancer. I don't expect one in my lifetime, though. Of course, we never know what's going to happen. I would hope so, but I don't expect it.

She had other hopes that were easier to describe. "What do I hope for right now? Just to be here. Just to be healthy for as long as the good Lord wants me to be here, and I pray that whatever I have to go through to make me strong. Give me the strength."

Throughout her experience with cancer, Mrs. Angel felt even more connected to God than she usually did. Her relationship with God was dynamic, with ups and downs, but always in constant contact and communication. She had always been a very religious woman. In her dining room hung a traditional portrait of Jesus, his expression exuding gentleness. Mrs. Angel's life was an attempt to be gentle like this Jesus and yet to fight aggressively enough to protect herself and stay alive. Lucille and her late husband, Mike, had both been active at their church. Mrs. Angel had been the secretary, and Mike had been a deacon. During Mike's illness their church attendance dwindled, and as he got sicker and the demands of caring for him grew, it ceased entirely. Mrs. Angel never felt comfortable going back to church after he died. After his death she became angry with God. She would seethe with anger whenever she thought about the criminal activity that regularly took place on the streets in front of her house. "My Mike is laying over there in Crown Hill, and these criminals get to go on living," she would complain. She was never able to reconcile this apparent injustice, and it was the basis for her anger. This anger also became its own form of torment, as she felt both shame and guilt because of it.

These feelings added another tension to her life and intensified her struggle. The conflict was between her anger at God and her view of herself as a faithful person. She suffered this privately and never rejoined her congregation as an active member, although she longed for a visit from her pastor. In fact, one day just before Christmas I visited and found her smiling from ear to ear. "I ran into my pastor, and he's going to come and see me," she explained. When I commented on the apparent importance of this to her, she replied, "You know how important church has always been to me." A few minutes later in a conversation about her separation from her congregation, I asked her if she thought her pastor should have made this offer before. She immediately replied, "Oh, yes. He's a man of God, isn't he?" For reasons I cannot stipulate with certainty, December came and went, as did January, February, March, April, May, and June, and Mrs. Angel's pastor never made his promised visit. Thus, she faced her crisis of faith alone in her prayers.

Despite her exile from church, Mrs. Angel never doubted her faith in God. She did, however, maintain a persistent anger toward Him. Her first husband, who had beaten her, was still living, while her second, loving husband was dead. She continued to stare out the window of her house and witness crimes being committed, pondering why her beloved husband, a good man, lay dead in his grave less than a mile away. She also wondered why she was being afflicted with cancer:

> I was angry at God when I lost my husband. I was angry then, and I was angry when I found out that I had cancer. . . . I was angry at myself, and I was angry at everybody and everything, but I prayed and asked the Lord to just remove that anger from me, you know, and help me be strong enough to deal with what I'm dealing with. And the Lord answers prayers, slowly but surely . . . he will answer your prayers. And that was one prayer he did answer for me.

Although she claimed to be over her anger, she was actually filled with ambivalent feelings. She said, "Eventually I'm going to get over this anger." She wondered if she was being punished in some way.

> What did I do? Did I do something to cause this to happen? I don't know what the reason is, but I know there's a reason for it. I pray a lot. First, I was asking the Lord to give me a reason, like I had done something wrong. I prayed, and I asked the Lord if he would forgive me. I don't think it's something I've done wrong. I don't think it is. It's just a part of life, I guess.

Despite her ambivalences, her connection with God through prayer remained constant, and she felt this gave her the strength to face what lay ahead. "Prayer is the main thing . . . when there's nothing else to do, prayer works—and God answers prayers."

Mrs. Angel and her daughter Rowanda talked through their feelings about God during this illness, growing closer because of these moments of shared spiritual intimacy. Rowanda said

> There's a lot of things that happen in our lives that we won't get an answer to. We know that God is good and God is love and God is always with us no matter what we're going through, and that he's not going to give us no more than we can bear. Even though we lost Papa, you had a stroke, and you were diagnosed with cancer all within a year's time, still God has not given us no more than we can bear, because we're still living on day to day.

Her mother answered:

> That's true. He won't give us any more of a burden than we can handle. The Lord is not going to put any more of a load on us to carry than he has to . . . no more. There's a reason for everything.

Although Mrs. Angel was clearly grieving in many ways, she still considered each day of her life a gracious gift from God. "Now, I can sit here teary-eyed and all this stuff and I feel sorry for myself sometimes, but then I look around. Since I've been coming back and forth to the hospital and doctors' offices, I had a chance to look around and see people sick, and I feel that I'm blessed compared to a lot of other people." Mrs. Angel often made connections with others in doctors' offices and in the hospital. "They always say, 'We are going to pray for you, Ms. Angel.' I say, 'Thank you, honey, I'm going to pray for you, too.' And I do. I don't forget those people."

Still, being sick made Mrs. Angel dwell on her own condition more than she thought was appropriate. "I didn't mean to sit up here and complain about God. God is the reason that I'm here, and he is a good God, too." She felt a vague uneasiness about discussing her feelings at such length. "I don't want to be a 'me, me' person. I never was a 'me, me' person, not every word that comes out of my mouth has got to be me and concern my sickness. I'm not that type of person. I don't want to be that type of person." She continued,

> At the first of every dawn I thank him for the beginning of another
> day starting in my life. . . . I don't wake up with the thought of,
> "Oh, Lord, I got cancer." I don't do that. I wake up and I thank the
> Lord for seeing me through the night and enabling me to see the
> beginning of another day. I wake up in the morning just thankful
> to be here and lay there in the bed.

Mrs. Angel deeply loved her three daughters. She tried to raise them to care for
one another and to be morally good people. Although her final battle with cancer
provided new opportunities for closeness, it also strained the bonds of motherhood
and sisterhood. One of Mrs. Angel's first thoughts when she discovered she had
cancer was about what it might do to her family. She received her diagnosis in
March, the final month of Mike's life. She was caring for him at home at the time,
and she decided not to tell her husband or the kids about her diagnosis. She did not
want him to have to worry about her, and she knew if she told the children they
would tell their papa. Consequently, this courageous and loving woman made the
decision to bear the burden of her diagnosis privately as a gift of love to her dying
husband.

After Mike's death she told her children she was concerned about them. "I was
worried about how they were going to handle this thing, this whole process. I was
not actually worried about myself, I was thinking of my family, how they were going to handle it." At first it drew her daughters to her side. One of the three would
always be with her for doctors' appointments and chemotherapy infusions. They
would come to her house on the weekends and help with shopping, cooking, and
cleaning. "We'd all just enjoy each other's company and everything, like when
they were at home." Rowanda was considering moving to Indianapolis from
Evansville to help her, but they had not yet decided if that was necessary.

They claimed they had open and honest relationships in which everyone felt
comfortable talking about any subject. "That was one thing good that came out of
that first marriage. My children and I are so close. We can sit down and talk to each
other, communicate with each other, about anything." Claims to total honesty
were exaggerated, as I will show, but there was an openness with which Mrs. Angel
and her daughters talked about painful topics. In the early stages after her diagnosis, no one dwelled on the subject of dying. "We don't talk about dying. I mean, if
the girls want to talk to me about it then they know I've always been there for them
and they've been there for me . . . we're just making plans to live."

Part of those plans involved planning for the holidays. As noted in Chapter 2,
Thanksgiving and Christmas were important traditions in Mrs. Angel's life, and
this was the first year since she married Mike that he would not be with them. Maintaining normalcy during this time was paramount. "We planned Thanksgiving and
we got plans for Christmas. We've always planned ahead of time, and I don't see
any reason to stop planning. That was the reason for the holiday dinner, Thanksgiving dinner, a big huge dinner, turkey and all the fixin's."

Unfortunately, a demon from the Angels' family past returned during Mrs. Angel's illness. Her youngest daughter, Joleen, and Joleen's daughter did not come to the family's Thanksgiving celebration. At first they speculated about where she had been, and her absence was blamed on sibling rivalry between Joleen and Tawana. "I don't know where she went for Thanksgiving. She wouldn't come home because her sister was here." Tawana left Indianapolis and returned home early on the holiday weekend so that Joleen could come home. This rivalry and conflict was immensely distressing to Mrs. Angel, who was trying to bring them back together:

> They're sisters, all three of them are sisters and like I told them, I carried all three for nine months under my heart and I gave birth to all three of them and I love all three of them. It just hurts me to see them getting along like this, and not coming together.

Apparently, Joleen's problems with Tawana had started in grade school and were undoubtedly related to the family problems they experienced while growing up. Their antagonisms occasionally erupted in physical fights, even as adults. Mrs. Angel did not want her daughters to reconcile because of her illness, but she was willing to try a bit of manipulation to get them to talk to each other. "I told my girls, which was a lie, but I told them, 'If this family cannot come together by Christmas, I will never ever have another family gathering at this house.'" When Rowanda argued that Mrs. Angel was not being fair to herself by making that threat, she continued, "If this family does not come together come Christmas, and I told them a lie, I said, 'I'm going to move to Ohio with my sister Denise.'"

It turned out that the issues involving Joleen ran deeper than sibling rivalry. Joleen had once been addicted to crack cocaine, and she began using drugs again while Mrs. Angel was sick. Joleen and her daughter moved in with Mrs. Angel for a brief period after Thanksgiving. It was difficult financially because the three of them were living on Mike's pension, but, as Mrs. Angel said, "God only knows I didn't mind them, because I could stretch it."

Mrs. Angel recognized later that Joleen had come to her house to try to save herself from her drug addiction. "Three weeks straight, she wasn't going out. She wouldn't go anywhere by herself, as if she thought, 'If I stay here with Mama, I'll be okay, right under Mama.'" Mrs. Angel knew she was free of drugs those three weeks. Then Joleen asked her mother if she could go out. Mrs. Angel told her, "You're grown. You don't have to ask me if it's okay, just be careful."

Joleen apparently began taking drugs again at that time and crossed the line of acceptable behavior in her mother's house. After accompanying Mrs. Angel to cash Mike's pension check, Joleen stole money from her mother for drugs while she was sleeping. "I was so hurt and upset. I said, 'How could you do this to me?' She couldn't explain it," Mrs. Angel lamented. Joleen offered to pay her mother back with her sixteen-year-old daughter's money. Mrs. Angel said, "No, you won't. That's her money. You're going to steal from her to pay me?" Then Mrs. Angel asked Joleen why she should not call the police, and Joleen began to cry. Mrs. Angel continued, "You either leave my house right now on your own, and when you go you make sure you take everything that belongs to you because you cannot come back in the house no more. Make sure you take everything that belongs to you right now. If you don't, I'll call the police." Joleen and her daughter left the house. Afterward, regret, guilt, and incessant worry about Joleen and her daughter began to eclipse all of Mrs. Angel's worries, including those about her own illness, and assumed much of her energies. "I got a call from the school the other day, my granddaughter had not been going to school. I don't know where they are. I feel as if I did it."

After her problems with Joleen, Mrs. Angel alternated between feeling angry and indignant and feeling guilty and loving. "For one of my children to do something like this to me and know what's going on. . . . I lost all trust in her. I'll never trust her." Seconds later she added, "I'll never stop loving her, because it's not her. This thing she did wasn't her. It's so unlike her. People talk to me and say when people get strung out on that drug, it'll make them do anything. And I believe it now." She also worried extensively about their safety, bemoaning how dangerous the streets were and "wondering what Joleen was getting into."

A large part of Mrs. Angel's efforts to come to terms with Joleen's problems focused on problems the family had faced growing up. She and Rowanda tried to make sense of Joleen's current problems. Mrs. Angel said, "She brings up a lot of things . . . childhood things. That makes sense." Rowanda pushed her, telling her that everyone else had resolved their issues related to those early years, and it was Joleen's turn to do the same. Rowanda said, "Our childhood was not all that great, but our childhood was not all that bad, either, because our childhood could've been a whole lot worse than what it was. Only by the grace of God that it didn't go that bad. If me and Tawana can come out of it and understand, Joleen should."

Although Rowanda placed much of the responsibility for Joleen's drug problems on Joleen's own shoulders, she also strove to be a mediator between her sister and mother. "It hurts her that Mama is sick, you know. It hurts her. . . . I ain't trying to protect Jo, I ain't trying to take up for her. But Jo's got to grow. We all got to go through our own thing, you know. But she does love Mama, and Mama loves Jo, and Mama also knows that Joleen is there for Mama and she hurts when Mama hurts. But she's just got another problem on the other end." Mrs. Angel, again vacillating between anger and pity, answered, "We've all got problems. Joleen has a problem that she can do something about and get herself straight. I got a problem, and all I can do is live with it."

After that conversation Mrs. Angel reflected on the events of her daughters' childhoods. This became a major source of stress and depression as well as a source of constant worry that exacerbated the suffering of the past year's tribulations. Three weeks later she was ready to talk about it again with her daughters. Joleen had been in touch with Rowanda. Mrs. Angel was relieved to know that Joleen and her daughter were safe. Joleen would not come to see her mother because she felt too ashamed. Rowanda told her, "She'll be in touch when she can bring herself to come and ask forgiveness for what she did." Mrs. Angel said, "Well, I'm glad. I've already forgiven her."

During these traumatic months Mrs. Angel often talked about Joleen as a child. "She was this little bitty kid, and she was just so loving. She just sort of clinged to me, you know, and said, Mommy, you know when you die, if you die Mom, I'm going to die too, Mama." At this point Mrs. Angel brought out a picture of Jo in the 1970s, when she was seventeen or eighteen years old. On the back was written, "To a person who I think could make my life worth living." Mrs. Angel said, "For her to say something like this at that age, it would mean to me that at that particular time there wasn't much to her life." She compared it to what was written on the back of a picture of Jo at age fourteen: "Ms. Joleen Jasmine Powell, age 14, 1733 Peach. Best-looking chick in E-town, right-on!"

In addition to trying to mediate between her two sisters and between her mother and Joleen, Rowanda also faced a dilemma with her father. As mentioned earlier, he had left the family and started a new family in Oklahoma. Apparently, he abused this family, too. He returned to Kentucky when he learned he was losing his sight due to glaucoma, but his two sisters would have nothing to do with him because he had abused them as well. Having nowhere else to turn, he "went to one of his children that he had walked off and left years ago, and Rowanda took him in."

All these family issues were occurring while Mrs. Angel's body was in rapid decline. The deficits from her stroke had worsened, and her mobility was increasingly impaired. She had become so weak that it was difficult for her to move from room to room. Her tumors were rapidly spreading, causing fatigue and difficulty in breathing. Nonetheless, she sought to take control of what she could. Secretly, in conjunction with me, she worked on funeral arrangements. Ever the caretaker, Mrs. Angel knew how hard her death would be on her daughters, and she wanted to spare them the burden of arranging the funeral. In the final three months of her life, a contest emerged between Mrs. Angel and her daughters revolving around the children's suspicions of what she was doing and her concealment of her funeral plans. In the end she arranged all the details of the viewing, services, and burial. Her children were eventually thankful, for it was one less form of stress they had to deal with during such a difficult time. It was also one final expression of Mrs. Angel's great love for them.

Mrs. Angel's condition worsened significantly during the last three months of her life. She became increasingly weak, and during the final month she was confined to her bed. She was so weak from her cancer and her previous stroke that she could not open a bottle of beer, which she enjoyed so much, so her son-in-law secretly opened several bottles of Budweiser and tucked them behind her pillow so she could drink them without her daughters' knowledge. This became a secret and important bond between the two of them.

Mrs. Angel was living in the shadow of death. In addition, she had endured enormous worry and consternation over Joleen and felt deeply guilty about the childhoods all her children had suffered. She was internally conflicted about many things: anger at God and guilt because of her anger; humiliation over the devolution of her body and shame over her vanity; anger at Joleen and guilt over throwing her out of the house; and deep disappointment over the abandonment by her pastor and congregation while struggling to remain nonjudgmental about others. Mrs. Angel suffered this turmoil privately and without the active support of shared religious rituals. Also, she endured this struggle, month after month, without the mindful presence of caring others from her congregation who might have offered a listening ear and shoulder to lean on. Despite this suffering, made even more acute by a sense of social isolation, she sought joy in life and actively sought comfort in God. Her daughters throughout these months were playing out, in their conflict with one another, issues that were unresolved from their childhood. Rowanda and Tawana were angry at Joleen. Joleen was angry with her mother. As Joleen confided, she was not just angry about the past, she was fearful and angry that "Mama was going to die." Running away to the streets was a way of evading the pain of her past and the imminence of her mother's death. In the final analysis, most difficult of all

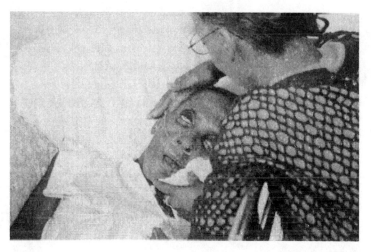

The daughters organized a symphonically coordinated twenty-four-hour vigil of caretaking, with each in charge of one eight-hour shift a day.

for each of the children was to watch Mrs. Angel deteriorate before their eyes and to know that the end of her life was approaching rapidly.

Her disease was progressing rapidly, and three days before her death Mrs. Angel slipped into a coma. She was uncommunicative, although her eyes were open, rolling back in her head. She was emaciated, and her body twitched. Later, her internal medicine physician told me that the cancer had most likely metastasized to her brain. It was probably the cause of the twitching, and in all likelihood did not cause her any pain, nonetheless she appeared to be in tremendous agony. Mrs. Angel's anguished visage and body twitches made the entire process extremely difficult for her daughters to witness.

Rowanda, Tawana, and Joleen came together during this period in a way that fully fulfilled Mrs. Angel's wishes for them to "be together as sisters." They took control of the dying process and worked as a team. They moved into the house and organized all the tasks they felt needed to be done for their mother: the Bible needed to be read, pain medicine needed to be given every thirty minutes, Vaseline needed to be applied to her lips, prayers needed to be said, baths needed to be given, and her hair needed to be brushed. They devised a chart, and when each task was done a small square was checked off. They divided each day into eight-hour shifts, with one of them in charge of a shift each day. In this way they were able to provide their mother with care and nurturing twenty-four hours a day. They touched her gently and prayed for her. Rowanda told her mother,

> **God is working this out, Mama. He's going to give you peace, real peace. He's going to give you rest, Mama, real rest. God is working this out for you, Mama, He's working it out. Keep the faith, Mama, your faith is strong. Keep your faith, Mama.**

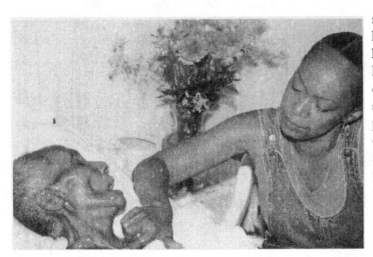

Rowanda says goodbye to her mother.

Mrs. Angel finally received a visit from her pastor the day before she died. She had been waiting eight months. Despite his unfulfilled promise, he was graciously welcomed into the home. Appearing uneasy at first and struggling to make eye contact, he asked everyone to leave the room in which Mrs. Angel was dying and prayed with her for two to three minutes. He came out of the room and shook the hands of her three daughters, her sister, and me. As he shook each hand he said, "All is well." He left approximately ten to fifteen minutes after he had arrived.

On the final day of her life, it seemed as if Mrs. Angel died fifty times. Her breathing was very labored. It would stop, and it would seem as if she were dead. Then it would resume. Her body was skin and bones. Her wig was off, and her hair was growing back in. Mrs. Angel died at home in her bed on July 13, 1999. Crying and with palms uplifted, Tawana prayed:

> My Mama is gone, oh Jesus, thank you. Dear Jesus, you are so
> good. I know you are so good. The seed was planted a long time
> ago. Thank you, dear Jesus.

The daughters first took turns saying goodbye at the bedside. After about fifteen minutes, they gathered in the kitchen to talk. They emerged a few minutes later to ask me to close their mother's eyes, saying that she had closed Mike's eyes after he died, and they knew it was important to her. They felt that they could not close them, so I told them it would be my privilege. Because her eyes had been straining toward the back of her head for some time, it was very difficult to get the eyelids to remain closed. As I tried several times, the daughters prayed, cried, and thanked God. They made promises that they would live from that moment on as sisters. Rowanda declared, "This is where the love started, with Mama. Now it's up to us to pass it on through our children and grandchildren." It took twenty minutes to get her eyes to stay shut. It was a time of great pain for her daughters, but it was also a sacred experience that they shared.

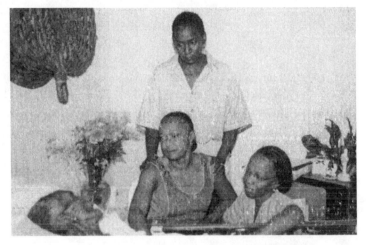

Three daughters brought together at the deathbed.

The three daughters then began a flurry of activities to distract themselves. Tawana began sweeping and cleaning. Rowanda talked about starting to cook a pot of chili. People from the neighborhood began to wander in. Dr. Lipton made a condolence call to the family after I contacted her. Hospice was called, and their community representative came to the Angel house.

After Mike had died, the funeral home had taken four hours to pick up the body. The stressful memory of that experience made the daughters anxious as they waited for the funeral home to pick up their mother's body. They made two frantic phone calls to see what was happening before the body was picked up about ninety minutes later. Her body was wrapped, placed in a bag, and removed on a stretcher. The daughters followed her out of the house and watched painfully as she was loaded into the mortuary's van and driven off.

Shortly thereafter they returned inside the house and decided they should begin calling everyone who had known their mother. They pooled their calling cards and began calling around the country. Rowanda stated that she was "going to keep calling until the Man gets angry with me." They ran up bills they could not afford to pay. All their phones were subsequently disconnected, and it was more than nine months later before they all had service again.

Mrs. Angel had a traditional Baptist funeral service three days later. She had a lovely coffin that was open for full viewing. About 100 people attended. The pastor declared at one point, "We all have to do this. We're all going to have to die." Her body was buried next to Mike's. Eighteen months later her children are still saving for a gravestone that they hope to be able to afford in about six more months.

Her children still grieve her loss. Rowanda is still caring for her father in Evansville, and says she sometimes remembers all the pain when she lies down at night and then prays for hours to be able to sleep. She has trouble finding anyone to support her:

> There's no one here but myself and my father, and he doesn't understand. . . . I go to church, but there's no support there. . . . I need to do something. I called a support group here two times, but she never called me back. I really miss her. I haven't gotten to the good memories yet. I'm still thinking about Thanksgiving and Christmas and what that was like without her. Just her passing. I think about it all the time.

Indeed, the death of Mrs. Angel was a great loss, particularly to her daughters, but also to everyone with whom she came in contact. I hope her daughters find the strength to resume their lives and keep their families together. Along with Rowanda, I pray that Mrs. Angel's body and gentle soul will find rest, real rest, and peace, real peace.

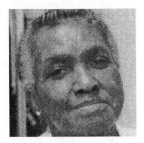

Chapter

6

LIFE ON THE BRINK:
MR. AND MRS. WHEELER

We have been cast aside, disregarded, and forgotten about.

—Bill Wheeler

Upon arriving at the home of Mr. and Mrs. Wheeler for the first time, I was enthusiastically welcomed. The house was a rental property on the near east side of the city. It was located in a racially mixed area that was relatively safe despite the fact that drug sales, street prostitution, and gang activity took place nearby. Most of the streets were fairly clean, but stray animals often roamed and lived on the neighborhood porches. The exteriors of the houses ranged from moderately good condition to downright disrepair. Overall, the neighborhood was dismal and lacking in aesthetic appeal. Obviously absent were flowers, ornamental trees, well-kept lawns, and other forms of landscaping that provide beauty and order in more affluent communities. Obviously present were chain-linked fences, older model cars parked in the streets, crowded semiattached houses, small front yards, and alleys spotted with dumpsters. There was also a lack of pedestrians, children playing in the streets or yards, and other forms of community interaction. Neighbors typically seemed uninvolved in one another's lives, tending to live in insular fashion without much connection to one another.

Entering the house for the first time, it was difficult not to be struck by its untidy condition. A disarray of dirty dishes filled the kitchen sink, spilling over onto the counter space. The walls throughout were stained, cracked, and dingy. There were no pictures or paintings to brighten their appearance. A large cockroach climbed a wall in the living room. Like the Whites, most striking in this dismal atmosphere was the fact that Mr. and Mrs. Wheeler spent a lot of their time at home without using indoor lights. Pressed by the financial demands of poverty, they restricted the use of lights to evening. The house was attached on one side and had another house located closely on the other side, leaving it naturally dark inside and allowing little opportunity for sunlight to enter. Because of economic constraints, the Wheelers spent a great deal of time sitting in relative darkness, typically alone. Like many inner-city poor, Judy and Bill used television as their main source of light, diversion, and connection to the world.

In stark contrast to the cheerless and gloomy circumstances in which the Wheelers lived was the hospitality they displayed. From the first visit, they always greeted me with remarkable ease and friendliness, often scurrying to turn lights on upon my arrival. Not only did this gracious attitude continue throughout our relationship, it blossomed into mutual respect and caring. Thus, from the beginning I was struck by the seeming discrepancy between the scarcity of their financial and material world and the abundant display of personal warm-heartedness they displayed.

The sincerity of their kindness was revealed right away. When I initially met them and explained this project, they were enthusiastic about participating. The overarching reason was altruistic. From the beginning Mr. Wheeler made his intentions clear:

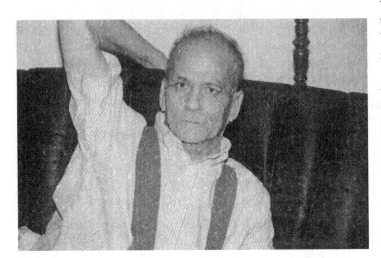

Enormous suffering lay ahead for Mr. Wheeler.

Yeah, I'll participate in your project. Maybe some good can come out of it. You know, not for me, but for others.

Very early on Mr. Wheeler let it be known that he was angry and mistrustful. He had grave misgivings about the public hospital system and was bitter and resentful about the care he received. He was convinced, with legitimate reason, that his illness had been misdiagnosed. He equally strongly believed he received "inferior care" because he had no health insurance.

Like so many indigent patients in the inner city, Mr. Wheeler used the emergency room (ER) of the public hospital as the front door to his primary health care. During the preceding two years he had been treated for gastrointestinal problems on multiple occasions in the ER. His care, like much that is rendered in this setting, was fragmented, lacked continuity, and was provided from the point of view of emergency medicine. Mr. Wheeler was never able to advocate successfully for a more comprehensive work-up than that provided in the context of emergency medicine. For most of that year, he continued, unfortunately, to rely on the emergency room for most of his health care. He also lacked the resources to become educated and empowered about his health and medical care. Faced with similar symptoms, most affluent persons would have greater success in accessing more comprehensive medical services. Not only would they have a wider array of choices, they would also be more likely to become self-educated about their condition. Libraries, bookstores, and the Internet, however, were not part of the world that Mr. Wheeler inhabited. To the contrary, his life was characterized by feelings of disempowerment and the absence of personal and economic resources. The sad result for Bill was that he wound up being diagnosed very late in the course of his illness and consequently had little chance of being helped by oncological intervention.

There can be no doubt that Mr. Wheeler was angry and embittered. This anger, however, was entirely internalized or expressed only to his wife. Neither he nor his wife were able to tell his doctors that they were dissatisfied and felt mistreated, nor were they able to articulate their wishes on how they wanted diagnosis and prognosis information communicated. The result was that they remained dissatisfied by what they were told and the manner in which important news was disclosed to them. The ironic fact is that, despite their discontent, they acted submissively in their interactions with their physicians, thus yielding to their authority while simultaneously being resentful of it. A tragic tension developed between their utter dependency on the technical skills and knowledge of physicians and their mistrust of the doctors upon whom they were so dependent.

Mr. Wheeler first became aware that he had cancer in late summer of 1998. He had been admitted to the hospital after a visit to the emergency room precipitated by raging stomach pain. A full battery of tests was conducted. On the day he received this life-altering diagnosis his wife had been with him for most of the afternoon. As luck would have it, however, she left a scant five minutes before the oncologist came into the room to inform him of the results of the tests that had been conducted, tests that revealed he had stomach cancer. Mr. Wheeler received the shocking news alone and remained alone to digest it after the oncologist left.

DAVID: *When you found out you had cancer, you were alone?*

MR. WHEELER: *Uh-huh . . . the cancer doctor came down and told me.*

MRS. WHEELER: *He was in the hospital.*

MR. WHEELER: *Yes, I was in the hospital. He came in and I started talking and I say, "Well what's wrong" and he says, "You got cancer" cause I told him not to hee-haw around it.*

DAVID: *So, he was straightforward?*

MR. WHEELER: *He was straightforward. Honesty is . . . that's always the best policy.*

DAVID: *Had you suspected that you might have cancer?*

MR. WHEELER: *No, I didn't. Yeah, it was very shocking . . . [and] I say "What?" And, he says, "You got cancer." And I say, "Well, how long?" And, he says, "I don't know."*

MRS. WHEELER: *They still haven't figured that out yet.*

MR. WHEELER: *He said, "You can take the treatment and they could cure it, and you could take treatments and it not help you at all." So, I says "Well, let's go for the treatments. That's the chance."*

DAVID: *Did hearing the news of having cancer scare you?*

MR. WHEELER: *Yeah, it did at first.*

MRS. WHEELER: *When I found out about it I was shocked. I think I was standing up and I had to go sit real quick.*

MR. WHEELER: *So, I just decided on the treatments and see what happens. Well, the first treatment that they gave me . . . the piece that they took out for the biopsy was as big as a golf ball . . . out of my neck.*

MRS. WHEELER: *I'm the one who told him about those lumps. I told the doctor about the knot in his neck. I said, "You need to check that out and see what this is," because it just kept getting bigger and bigger.*

MR. WHEELER: *And, uh . . . you can feel it now and there are just small knots there. And these was, you know like I said, as big as golf balls.*

A lot is going on here. Mr. Wheeler had received devastating news, news that he seemed surprised and unprepared to hear. The news was delivered to him in isolation, and that exacerbated his initial anxieties. In a twenty-minute conversation his life had been transformed, and he had much to think about. Not only was he trying to comprehend the bad news, he had to decide how and when to tell his wife. He chose not to call her and disclose the diagnosis over the phone. Rather, he elected to wait until the next day. During this period of time he tossed and turned emotionally over two things. The first was anxiety related to hearing the diagnosis. As he tells it, his head "was swimming with all kinds of worries." The second concern was what to tell his wife. At first he toyed with the idea of not telling her at all but came to the conclusion that that would be unfair. As Mr. Wheeler recollects, telling her was important, "the only way to go." Nonetheless, the short-term agony of deciding how and what to tell her was a burden imposed by the fact that he had been informed about the cancer without her being present.

MR. WHEELER: *He seemed like he's like, you know, a caring doctor. He says, "Is there anybody down here smoking or somebody here with you today?" And I said, "My wife just left to go. She just did leave about five minutes ago."*

DAVID: *Would you rather have had her there with you?*

MRS. WHEELER: *I would rather I had been there. Yeah, I could have asked questions and stuff.*

DAVID: *How about you, Mr. Wheeler, would you rather she had been there?*

MR. WHEELER: *Well, yeah. Yes and no. At first I wasn't going to tell her. I went around and around in my mind all the rest of the day and that night about not telling her. I says, "No, that's cheating her." And I didn't ever cheat on her or cheated her before and I wasn't going to this time. So, I told her the next morning.*

DAVID: *So, you had a truth-telling session?*

MR. WHEELER: *Yep.*

DAVID: *In the hospital?*

MR. WHEELER: *Well, outside in the smoking area.*

MRS. WHEELER: *When I came up to him, he had this bad look on his face, and I was wondering what was wrong.*

MR. WHEELER: *If I had told her anything else, she'd known I was lying.*

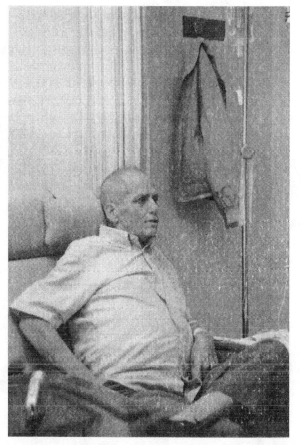

Opting for experimental chemotherapy, Mr. Wheeler remained deeply resentful of the doctors on whom he was so dependent.

I realize that it goes against the grain of institutional efficiency, but perhaps no one should ever be told of a serious, life-threatening diagnosis while alone unless that is his or her explicit wish. It seems that the doctor missed an opportunity by not asking Bill if a chaplain might join them for the discussion. One can only imagine the inner angst and turmoil he experienced after the oncologist left, how hearing the very word *cancer* brought dark and frightening images to his mind, how the fear of dying—of being slowly annihilated by cancer—"swam" in his head, and how he worried about what this meant for the future and how much he was going to suffer before it was all over—one way or another. These were the thoughts that raced through his mind as he restlessly slept that night, fear and worry stabbing at his heart. In many ways the unrest of these first twenty-four hours established a pattern of turmoil from which

he would never escape. From this point on Mr. Wheeler remained emotionally dismantled and battled his cancer in constant and unrelieved agitation.

Conversely, the resilience of his spirit, even in the face of having received the unexpected and horrible news of a cancer diagnosis, was striking. Although Mr. Wheeler
would never know normal life again and would experience precious little joy in the year
to come, he did find the strength within to bear the burden of his diagnosis. Although
his mind and emotions were overwhelmed, he expressed gratitude at the straightforward demeanor of his doctor. Additionally, he came to a practically and morally sound
decision about telling his wife. In his unique way Mr. Wheeler came to the conclusion
that loyalty, faith-
fulness, and perhaps
practicality de-
manded that he be
honest with her.
From this point on,
their relationship
would never be the
same. Illness, suffer-
ing, and dying would
transform their part-
nership and generate
deep hardship but
also create a bond of
intimacy that they
had never been able
to achieve while
healthy.

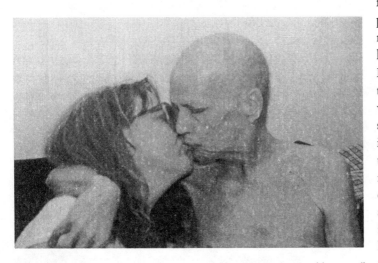

"Had it not been for this cancer, we would have been divorced by now,"
said Bill Wheeler.

The "diagnosis
conversation" was
also a choice point. It established the path Mr. Wheeler would take during the next
year of his life. Remember that he was told that he "could take the treatment and
possibly be cured." Actually, the fact of the matter was that he was being instructed
that if he wanted to live chemotherapy was his only choice, period! Something
very subtle, yet profound, was happening. Technological intervention was being
introduced as a potential lifesaver, his only possible savior. He made the decision to
accept treatment, and as a result procedures, tests, and medical information became
predominant in the end-of-life experience for both him and his wife. In their fear
and vulnerability, they quickly became dependent on chemotherapy. They saw it as
a reason for hope. This technical–medical focus also provided a safe haven for his
doctors. By focusing their attention on clinical matters they could avoid the moral
and emotional messiness of the "big issue" of dying and concentrate on treating
his disease and symptoms.

Chemotherapy initially provided a hopeful refuge for Mr. and Mrs. Wheeler. Through it they were able to believe, at least for a while, that he would be cured. Later, they felt let down and disillusioned when it became clear that the chemotherapy was not working. When they finally came to recognize that he was going to die, they painfully realized that there had never been a realistic chance of cure in the first place. As a result they became even more disillusioned, angry, and mistrustful. An important moral and ethical issue is raised here, one that is very common to the practice of medicine in treating advanced illness. It has to do with the importance of hope, which, as noted in Chapter 2, is critical. However, the Wheelers' narrative also points to the dangers of false hope, which not only intensifies suffering in the long run but also is a breeding ground for resentment, anger, and diminished quality of life.

Although Mr. Wheeler was shocked to hear that he had cancer, he had not felt well for quite some time. He had lost 100 pounds over the course of several months. In fact, when he showed me a picture that had been taken a few years earlier, I was stunned at the transformation. He truly was a mere shadow of his former self.

MR. WHEELER: *When I first started losing weight I didn't know what was going on. I was going to Dr. Lens at the time, wasn't I?*

MRS. WHEELER: *You saw Dr. Jones.*

MR. WHEELER: *And he gave me them stomach pills. That's why I said I didn't know if I asked him or not. That other guy. Uh, but he gives me them stomach pills and they did help for a long time, didn't they?*

MRS. WHEELER: *Uh-huh.*

MR. WHEELER: *And uh . . . they quit working. When I lost the weight, like I said a minute ago, everything was off, I guess. Only took about three months.*

DAVID: *Three months to lose 100 pounds?*

MR. WHEELER: *Yep . . . It was just like peeling a banana. Taking the peelings off a banana I just lost it that fast.*

MRS. WHEELER: *You kept telling me that "I think there is something wrong with my stomach these doctors won't tell me."*

MR. WHEELER: *Yes, I told her that there was something wrong with my stomach.*

MRS. WHEELER: *He kept on telling the doctors his stomach was hurting and they didn't pay any attention. They just let it go in one ear and out the other. It kept on getting worse and worse.*

MR. WHEELER: *I knew there was something wrong.*

This experience was particularly important to Mr. Wheeler. He wanted this part of his story told loud and clear. In his view if he had not been an indigent, uninsured patient in the public hospital system, he would have had more diagnostic tests run earlier in his illness. Mr. Wheeler lived with the distinct impression that being poor, being a patient in the public hospital, relying so heavily on the emergency room as his site of primary care, and receiving rushed care that lacked continuity when he would be seen at the primary care clinic were the factors that would ultimately cost him his life. In his view the culprit was much less his cancer than it was the inadequate care he received.

Very quickly, consistent with the private expectations of his doctors, his disease progressed and brought significant physical decline and serious life restrictions. He sighed deeply and with disgust, lamenting what the cancer was doing to him.

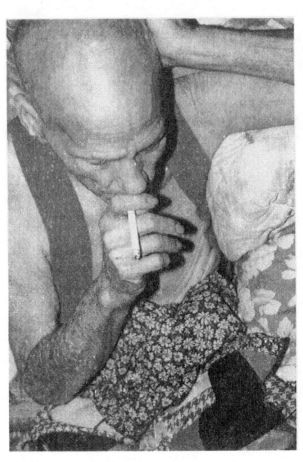

Disease is rapidly progressing.

MR. WHEELER: *Now, I am just here . . . just here. How am I going to put it? No energy? Used to be before I got sick it'd be hard to catch me at home. I'd be down on the creek bank fishing or pay lake or fishing somewhere. This year we ain't went.*

MRS. WHEELER: *He said we were going fishing a lot this year, but we couldn't.*

MR. WHEELER: *When you are this sick you don't feel like going out and sitting on the creek bank.*

MRS. WHEELER: *You used to like to go outside and, you know, sit outside. But now, anymore he's in the house.*

Not only was Mr. Wheeler becoming increasingly sequestered in his home, he was starting to feel "really lousy" most of the time. His stomach was in constant pain, which created distress for both Judy and him. As he commented, "I wished I'd feel a little bit better. See, like right now my belly is hurting again." Mrs. Wheeler added, "It stays that way. His belly hurts constantly anymore. I don't know what to do. I'm getting to where I don't know what to feed him." Simply put, he was feeling awful, both physically and emotionally, a feeling that would only grow in the months to come.

Compounding his physical decline, with its corresponding pain and emotional distress, was the deepening and relentless anger toward a system of care that he felt had failed him. Asked to describe his feelings, he spoke often of being "depressed" and "disgusted," depressed about a hideous disease that was destroying his body and disgusted by the sense of betrayal that he felt by a system of care on which he was utterly dependent:

> I want it [a healthy Mr. Wheeler] back! I tell you, like I have ever since last week. If people had insurance or got money, you get better care out there. I believe in that, and nobody's going to change my mind. 'Cause if it was some place else and you were complaining about your belly for three months, and you had insurance, they'd find out what was wrong with your belly.

Anger, mistrust, and deep feelings of abandonment shaped his psychoemotional state. In fact, they were his constant companions. Throughout the destruction of his body, his spirit and mind seemed inseparable from these negative feelings. Sadly for a man who wanted to live and clutch onto the joys of life so much, he found it next to impossible to enjoy "one day at a time." Throughout his illness he was never able to find a sense of peace within himself. During the first month after receiving his diagnosis, things got so bad that he flirted seriously with the idea of suicide. He would sit on the couch in the living room next to the table where he kept all his medicines. There, in the dark and in the fear that frequently took control of his mind, he would brood about ending his suffering by killing himself. "I thought about it real seriously," he said. "I wasn't sure I could cope. But Judy and I talked about it. We decided that we wanted to be together. Me and her talked it over, and we decided that life's better than that, and we'll just take one day at a time." At this point, for better or worse, Mr. Wheeler came to two conclusions: that he would fight against his cancer and that he would wage this battle rather than give up so he and Mrs. Wheeler could have "thirty more years together." Thus, despite being at the threshold of suicide, his desire for life prevailed:

MR. WHEELER: *Well, I'll tell you the truth. She went to bed one night I picked up the pills and had them in my hand. It wouldn't have took very long.*

DAVID: *What made you pull it back?*

MR. WHEELER: *Mrs. Wheeler.*

DAVID: *Did she come out?*

MR. WHEELER: *Nope. Just a little voice you know. Just "Don't do that." She knows when I am thinking shit.*

MRS. WHEELER: *I want him to live. To live for me and for his family . . . we only gonna be married two years and that's just too short.*

DAVID: *You feel ripped off?*

MRS. WHEELER: *No. I just don't want him to be like my other husband and die in front of me. I don't think I could stand it. Of course, I'll face it if I have to. But. . . .*

MR. WHEELER *(interrupting): I decided against it. The next morning I told her. I told her I am going to take one day at a time.*

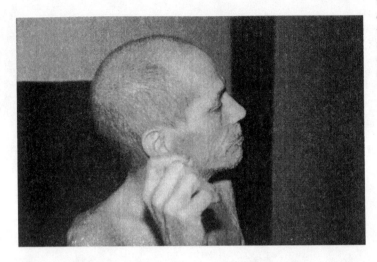

"Because with chemotherapy, you got at least halfway a chance, without it you don't. I don't know if I'd commit suicide or not then," Mr. Wheeler concluded.

In a whirlwind of worry, chaos, and contemplation of suicide, Mr. Wheeler made a conscious choice to embrace life. In doing so he became increasingly dependent on medical treatment. Simply put, Mr. Wheeler came to the conlusion that "life is better," his confrontation with mortality seemingly making it all the more precious. He often spoke with strong enthusiasm about his newly discovered consciousness of life and respect for the joys it offered. "Yeah, yeah. I desire life more now than ever before." He put this resurrected reverence for life in perspective:

> Well, I respect life on the account of you can't see birds fly if you are dead, you can't see 'em fly. You can't see the squirrels or nothin' if you're dead. When you are alive you can see all that stuff . . . and that's important. Like life, even the way the world is today, life's better than being dead.

Despite his yearnings for life's joys and pleasures, his daily existence was becoming more and more restricted by the battle against disease. The cancer was aggressively attacking his body, inflicting new levels of pain and suffering:

MR. WHEELER: *I don't like the pain and suffering, because, you know, it's hell to wake up with your body hurting and you feel like you are all drugged out especially when you have to take all of the medicine there. . . . So, I am in very much discomfort . . . yeah, on a scale of 1 to 10, a 10.*

DAVID: *Could you describe that pain?*

MR. WHEELER: *It was like something in there just eating away. Just right across the belly to the side and then goes to the back . . . I just cope with it. The steady ache. Uh, it's like uh, somebody pulling your teeth with no Novocain or nothing. I did use those pain pills, but I don't like to take them.*

MRS. WHEELER: *Tell him what your pain pills do.*

MR. WHEELER: *Well, I can take the pain pills if I have to, but I had to go to sleep all the time.*

Mr. Wheeler's reluctance to take the medicine to control pain was directly related to his newly developed regard for life. When asked why he would choose to suffer pain rather than take the medicine, he responded that it was important to remain alert and avoid being knocked out by the narcotics:

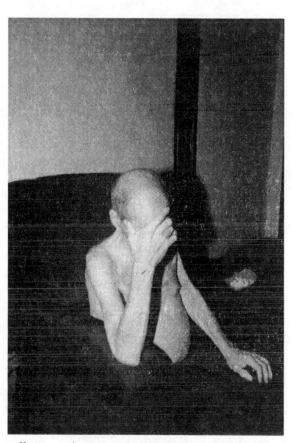

> I guess it's all about life. When you are asleep you do not know anything. So when you are awake you can look outside. If you feel halfway decent, you can step outside for a few minutes. If you're asleep, you can't do that.

Suffering and agony precipitate a recontemplation of suicide.

Ironically, in his struggle to live, Mr. Wheeler became more and more dependent on the system he so hated. Although continually resentful of his status as an indigent patient in the public hospital, he organized his life around medical information, procedures, and appointments. In his own way, he became proficient in navigating the bureaucracy. For example, he realized fairly quickly that scheduled appointments in the primary care and oncology clinics meant little. Typically, he would have to wait two to three hours, sometimes more, to be seen. Figuring out that the clinic essentially operated on a first-come, first-served basis despite scheduled appointments, he would arrive for an afternoon clinic appointment around 11:45 AM. He would have to wait more than an hour, but he would be first in line and be seen fairly promptly around 1:00 PM. In a very interesting way, his life was becoming intimately connected to and defined by a system that often incensed him. In this connection, he learned how to "play the game," part of which was to suffer his discontent quietly so as not to antagonize the people on whom he was reliant. Thus, despite enormous dissatisfaction with his care, Mr. Wheeler never expressed his displeasure. Disempowered in his interactions with his doctors, he sought other means of empowerment. One of these was finding ways to beat the bureaucracy at its own game.

At this point some very contradictory things began to happen. Consistent with the aggressiveness of his disease, his symptoms worsened. Consistent with his deepened appreciation of life, he became increasingly embittered by having to live with so much pain and discomfort. His distress became so severe that he began thinking, once again, that death might be preferable. Like most mortals would do if in his place, Mr. Wheeler began to ponder and question why he was suffering so much and if all this misery were somehow connected to God's plan. In this contemplation for the first time in his life he began to "wonder what the big picture is about." In this musing, Death (with a capital D) was no longer just an abstract concept but an impending reality. When asked to describe his thoughts about Death, he would speak in the same breath about how it would be a welcomed relief yet was something he feared and would fight against:

MR. WHEELER: *It has to be better than this.*

DAVID: *Death is better than this?*

MR. WHEELER: *Well, in a way, yes.*

DAVID: *How so?*

MR. WHEELER: *No pain. You don't have to worry about any pain. And you don't have to worry about your gas bills, your light bills, anything like that.*

We can only imagine how deeply Mr. Wheeler was suffering with the viselike grip of pain and discomfort overwhelming both his mind and spirit:

MRS. WHEELER: *His stomach is always hurting. It never stops hurting.*

MR. WHEELER: *Like right now, it's just roaring. . . . I think my cancer is still there because my belly hurts constantly. It hurts like it did at first, don't it?*

MRS. WHEELER: *It don't let up.*

MR. WHEELER: *They're going to have to do something, even with them pills, because them pills don't help any. I could take them around the clock and it wouldn't help.*

The burden of illness combined with the hardships of poverty were clearly taking their toll. His need for relief of myriad sufferings was so deep that it sometimes seemed to be stronger than his will to live, yet moments later in the same conversation his fighting attitude would resurface. In discussing how his mind was "swimming in different thoughts," which occurred more frequently as he felt sicker, Mr. Wheeler recommitted to "the battle." He spoke from the intensive care unit:

MR. WHEELER: *I have these thoughts . . . especially when like Friday, Saturday, I didn't think I was going to make it Saturday. Now I do. . . . I'm fightin' more today than I had all day Saturday.*

DAVID: *You didn't think you were going to make it Saturday, now you do?*

MR. WHEELER: *Uh huh, yes. . . . you know when you say you are not going to give up on something?*

DAVID: *Yes.*

MR. WHEELER: *That's the way I feel. I'm not going to give up. I'm not. . . . I'm going to fight it every step of the way. . . . Going to live every minute I can. I ain't gonna be stupid and take my life with something I can't control.*

DAVID: *I know you thought about that for a while.*

MR. WHEELER: *Yep.*

DAVID: *Are you glad you made that decision?*

MR. WHEELER: *Yeah.*

DAVID: *You told me a few minutes ago that death has to be better than this, because there will be no pain, there will be no suffering.*

MR. WHEELER: *Right.*

DAVID: *You have been through a lot in the past few months.*

MR. WHEELER: *Uh, huh. Stroke, heart attack. . . . See, I keep bouncing back.*

DAVID: *You have had a lot of nausea; a lot of pain.*

MR. WHEELER: *Lots of pain!*

DAVID: *Lots of pain. All of that was worth going through?*

MR. WHEELER: *Just to be with my wife. . . . if she wasn't a part of this I probably would have ended it.*

Despite literally being tortured by physical suffering and despondency, Bill remained strongly connected to his wife. It was this connection, revitalized in illness, that made him continue to choose life over suicide once again:

> What's going to hurt me is just leaving my wife. I could spend the next hundred years with her.

Thus, at least at this point, the tension between fighting cancer and giving up was resolved by his hope of spending more time with Judy, from whom he feared being separated.

There was increasing ambivalence in the world of Mr. Wheeler, ambivalence that was intensifying both his and Judy's confusion. Remember that he commented that he still thought his "cancer was there." This comment was made in reference to a conversation he had had several weeks earlier in the oncology clinic. This conversation, or more accurately "misconversation," with both the staff oncologist and the oncology fellow had led him to believe that he was in remission.

One Wednesday morning, several months into his chemotherapy regimen, I walked over to the oncology clinic to visit Mr. Wheeler with Dr. G. He excitedly greeted us, not just with enthusiasm but also with a smile. Smiling was out of the ordinary for Mr. Wheeler, so we quickly suspected something unusual was up. Before we could even exchange greetings, he exclaimed, "Guess what?" Not waiting for us to respond, he blurted out, "Remission!" His tone could not have been more emphatic or hopeful. Clearly, we were taken aback because we were aware of the clinical details surrounding the cancer and knew that his oncologists believed he was incurably ill. In fact, his oncologist referred him to the project precisely because he knew he was not going to make it, a factor made explicit by the comment, "I'm afraid we got him too late in his disease process to be of any help to him." This comment was made after the doctor saw Mr. Wheeler for the first time in the clinic. When I asked Bill to explain what was going on,

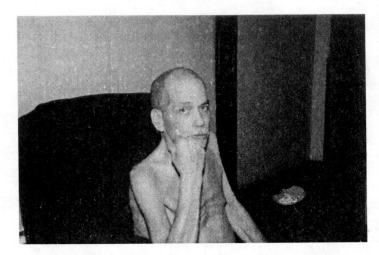

Still believing that he is "in remission and on the way to being cured."

he stated that the oncologist had told him that "the medicines were working" and that they were on their "way to remission and a cure." What followed was an awkward conversation. We asked Mr. Wheeler exactly what he had been told, what he understood remission to mean, and what he understood this meant for him. He was very straightforward in his answers. He had been told that he was responding favorably to the chemotherapy and that he was in remission, and that meant he was headed toward having his health restored.

In reality, something quite different was occurring. In a small way, Mr. Wheeler was responding unexpectedly and favorably to the chemotherapy. There had been some observable shrinkage in the lymph nodes in his neck. The oncologists seized on this isolated good news and focused their conversation on it with him. When Mr. Wheeler asked what this meant, they reassured him that if this response continued, he would be moving toward remission and cure. Mr. Wheeler, hearing the yearned-for words *remission* and *cure* focused his attention exclusively on them. In doing so, he misconstrued the conversation to mean that he was in remission, therefore becoming hopeful for complete cure. This misunderstanding was not only the fault of Mr. Wheeler's selective attention and focus. The physicians also shared a significant responsibility. Although they were surprised that his tumors were responding at all, they knew full well that his response was going to be only temporary. Introducing the prospect of remission and cure when they knew otherwise was misleading. They were well intentioned, as reported in Chapter 3, but misleading nonetheless. Despite offering short-term comfort, this conversation was ultimately injurious to both Mr. and Mrs. Wheeler.

As Mrs. Wheeler recalls, the doctors came into the treatment room, and the staff doctor said, "It looks like the medicine is doing what we want." On hearing the word *remission* she noted how much better it made her feel. "Like music to my ears. That gave me hope, you know, that does give you a lot of hope, when they say it is going into remission." When asked what it meant for him to hear the word, Mr. Wheeler responded that it was "damn good."

Mr. Wheeler became quite hopeful as a consequence of this conversation. The hope at first was real. In the beginning his wife, too, seemed to believe that he was in remission. Later, however, she confided that she always had a slice of doubt, as she just could not understand how someone who felt and looked so terrible could really be on the road

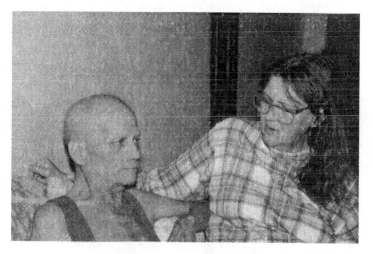

With illness and death continually facing her husband, Mrs. Wheeler struggled to maintain the belief that he was in remission.

to recovery. Nonetheless, in the beginning they both took comfort in the belief that he was in remission. Their faith in it became a way of coping with their stress and strain, at least for the short term. Even without knowing the clinical details, any casual observer who looked at Mr. Wheeler would have known that he was extremely sick and was not going to get better. From my own personal and professional perspective, along with the individuals who were assisting in the project, the picture was even more complicated and painful. Not only were we aware of the clinical details that made for a grim prognosis, we also knew that major miscommunication had occurred between the Wheelers and the oncologists. There was some strong opinion among us that we should get involved and help straighten out the situation. We worried about the negative impact when he would finally be told that he was not in remission, but was dying. I had no doubt that Bill would feel tumultuous disillusionment, which would be harmful for a man who already did not trust his doctors. Others, who did not know Mr. Wheeler but were part of the project team, felt that we would risk our professional reputations and relationships with doctors if we interfered in any way.

Frankly, the tension between the competing obligations of doing right by Mr. and Mrs. Wheeler versus not alienating his doctors created some internal conflict that was never satisfactorily resolved. In addition, it also revealed a fundamental and perhaps inevitable conflict in my role as observer, witness, and participant. As a purely objective observer, my purpose was to record the story as it happened. Inevitably, as a partnership with suffering patients and families developed, I became more than a disconnected onlooker to their stories. I became a witness to their sorrow and, consistent with the goal of becoming a voice for them, I also became a caring participant in their lives and deaths. In doing so, I became intimately connected with them and was able to witness parts of their lives that I would not have been able to see otherwise had I not been so close to, and therefore trusted by, them. Nonetheless, despite the value of building a close bond with patients and families, from time to time this involvement created moral dilemmas and sometimes inflicted guilt over not becoming involved in situations in which I believed I could be helpful.

The urgency of resolving the conflict about whether to respond to the misapprehensions of remission of the Wheelers was set aside because of an unexpected occurrence. Mrs. Wheeler was not only showing signs of stress from caring for her husband, she was beginning to feel ill. In addition to fatigue, her stomach had been hurting for several weeks, and she had lost about thirty pounds during the past three months. Her obstetrics/gynecology doctors ordered some tests and referred her to the hematology clinic. When I met her and Mr. Wheeler for the appointment, she immediately said, "He's no longer the only one who is really sick," referring to her husband. After a thirty-minute wait during which she fidgeted nervously while Mr. Wheeler remained stonily still, the hematologist entered the exam room and began:

DOCTOR: *I think we do not have absolute proof right now that the type of lymphoma we are dealing with is one of those slow-rolling, indolent lymphomas. The reason for this is because of the small amounts of tissue that they removed with the muscle biopsy.*

MRS. WHEELER: *Uh-huh.*

DOCTOR: *Unfortunately, it is good to tell us that you have lymphoma, but it is not good to tell us which type of lymphoma you have. Okay? You see my point?*

MRS. WHEELER: *Yes.*

DOCTOR: *Do you have any lumps?*

MRS. WHEELER: *No.*

DOCTOR: *You don't have any lumps, okay.*

MRS. WHEELER: *The doctor hasn't said anything about it.*

DOCTOR: *Well, I'll find out. If you have a lump in your neck that would be the best thing.*

MRS. WHEELER: *Yeah, like I do.*

DOCTOR: *That would be the best way to go. I mean, if you don't, we may have to discuss between me and you what to do next to get a better piece of tissue to make a diagnosis of this lymphoma. . . .*

MRS. WHEELER: *Uh-huh.*

DOCTOR: *Okay, now the reason for that is not trivial because that will change dramatically what we are going to do. If we prove that this is one of those lymphomas which are very indolent . . . then we are fine. On the other hand, if during the biopsy through the operation we are going to find a lymphoma which is not as indolent as we thought just based on that little needle thing . . .*

MRS. WHEELER: *(interjecting): Uh-huh.*

DOCTOR: *That would be an indication to treat you, okay? Because the natural history that caused the lymphoma would be different, okay? So, all of this is coming really kind of fast, so I know that you need to have time to digest all this.*

MRS. WHEELER: *No.*

DOCTOR: *You don't?*

MRS. WHEELER: *No.*

DOCTOR: *Okay.*

MRS. WHEELER: *I'm understanding.*

DOCTOR: *Alright, very well.*

The conversation then shifted to a discussion of the details of the biopsy, that it would be three to four weeks before it could be performed, and that she would need to be in the hospital for a few days. Mrs. Wheeler proceeded to talk about her back problems and that she was seeing a gynecologist. After a brief discussion of estrogen replacement therapy, the doctor sought to bring the discussion to a close so he could begin his physical exam:

DOCTOR: *Okay, do you have any other medical problems except the ones you just mentioned?*

MRS. WHEELER: *My nerves, epilepsy.*

MR. WHEELER: *She's got real bad nerves.*

DOCTOR: *Bad nerves?*

MRS. WHEELER: *I'm seeing a psychiatrist for my nerves right now.*

DOCTOR: *Okay, alright. Why don't you come over here and lay down on the table.*

The doctor performed a very thorough physical exam and decided it was necessary to admit her to the hospital for the aforementioned biopsy. He unhurriedly discussed with her what it would entail—pain, discomfort, local anesthesia, and so on. He instructed that she would have to be patient with scheduling. Mrs. Wheeler was extremely anxious to find out exactly what was wrong, but in County Hospital there is always an extended wait for nonemergency procedures.

DOCTOR: *We have to wait until we get a date for the surgery, okay?*

MRS. WHEELER: *You have to get it down at surgery?*

DOCTOR: *Right.*

MRS. WHEELER: *I'll have to be in the hospital longer.*

DOCTOR: *We can do a biopsy probably here at County, but the scheduling is so tight. We are always running behind for that. We have no time to do this thing here. Okay?*

MRS. WHEELER: *Uh-huh. Alright. Thank you.*

The minute the doctor left the room, Mrs. Wheeler stated, "I don't want to go to the hospital." Her husband responded, "Well, he wants to be safe rather than sorry." She replied, "Oh." Overwhelmed by her own personal predicament but still worried about him, she asked, "Who is going to take care of you while I'm in the hospital?" "Me! I think I'm big and ugly enough," he reassured her.

The situation was getting more difficult by the day. For Mrs. Wheeler there was a nagging fear of pain. "I can't stand pain," she admonished her doctor in regard to the biopsy. Additionally, there was the fear of hospitals and procedures that she readily admitted intimidated and frightened her. Also, as she confided to me privately, she was worried that the course of her illness would parallel the path of steady decline that her husband had experienced over the past six months. She was profoundly anxious not just about her future but about what her illness would mean in terms of her capacity to care for him. Despite what she said to her doctor, she understood very little about what was going on. When I asked if she understood what kind of disease lymphoma is, she could offer no explanation other than "cancer." When I inquired if she understood what an "indolent lymphoma" is, she gave a puzzled look and simply said "No." When she was asked if she understood why surgery was not an option for her disease, all she could say was, "No, he just said he couldn't do it."

Once again, the point is that while uncertainty and disempowerment are normal in the illness experiences of all individuals, they are even more profound in the world of the dying poor. If one listens carefully to the interaction between Mrs. Wheeler and the hematologist, the degree of separation between their worlds becomes apparent.

Lacking education and ability to access educational resources that might have helped her become more knowledgeable and empowered, this gap would never be closed. Her only plausible option, as was the case with her husband, was to rely on her doctors and health-care providers, abiding by and resting in their decisions.

One week later Mrs. Wheeler had an appointment in the primary care clinic. Her primary care doctor, a first year medical intern, entered and began the conversation.

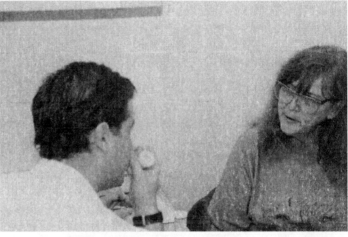

DOCTOR: *You are going to have to sit in the hot seat [he scooted a chair]. Okay. So catch me up, because I've been a little bit out of the loop as far as your diagnosis. What's been going on?*

MRS. WHEELER: *Well they was supposed to start workin' on me Thursday.*

DOCTOR: *Okay. So it's been a week from yesterday.*

MRS. WHEELER: *Yes.*

DOCTOR: *So, a week from yesterday you are going to have what?*

More chaos, medical uncertainty, and dependency on doctors define the world of Mrs. Wheeler.

MRS. WHEELER: *Hematology.*

DOCTOR: *An appointment?*

MRS. WHEELER: *Yes.*

DOCTOR: *And what is the process of diagnosis so far?*

MR. WHEELER: *Cancer.*

MRS. WHEELER: *It's cancer.*

DOCTOR: *I know we know it's a lymphoma, okay? Have the surgeons . . . have you talked to the surgeons?*

MRS. WHEELER: *I have not talked to nobody except for Dr. James.*

DOCTOR: *Dr. James, a hematologist?*

MRS. WHEELER: *He may be.*

DOCTOR: *I don't know all the names.*

MRS. WHEELER: *He's an oncologist. [In fact, he was a hematologist.]*

DOCTOR: *Okay.*

MRS. WHEELER: *I broke down, I said I'm getting tired of waiting. I want to find out now what is going on. Nobody tells me nothing.*

DOCTOR: *Okay.*

MR. WHEELER: *She had phone calls in . . . no returns.*

MRS. WHEELER: *I tried to get a hold of Sara because I needed her to let me know something.*

DOCTOR: *Sara . . . the ob/gyn?*

MRS. WHEELER: *Ob/gyn doctor.*

DOCTOR: *Yes.*

MRS. WHEELER: *She won't return my phone calls.*

DOCTOR: *I don't think that's like her.*

MRS. WHEELER: *No, it's not. I don't think it's like her either.*

DOCTOR: *Yeah, 'cause she returned all my phone calls, and I know she was close in touch with you. . . .*

MRS. WHEELER: *There for a while. . . .*

DOCTOR: *Right.*

MRS. WHEELER: *Then she went. . . .*

DOCTOR: *She went bye-bye.*

MRS. WHEELER: *Yes.*

DOCTOR: *Okay.*

DOCTOR: *Alright. So, we are dealing with a lot these days?*

MRS. WHEELER: *Yes, and . . . the main thing is my back. . . .*

DOCTOR: *Is that new? I don't remember you complaining about your back.*

MRS. WHEELER: *Well, my back is being out for some time. I've got two discs.*

DOCTOR: *Huh?*

MR. WHEELER: *It's been out for going on three years.*

DOCTOR: *Okay. Because . . . I think, so far, what we've talked about primarily, before this all crept up, was your nerves.*

MRS. WHEELER: *Uh-huh, my nerves are still bad. You have not yet got my appointment with that woman. . . .*

MR. WHEELER: *With a psychiatrist.*

DOCTOR: *A psychiatrist . . . um, I'm pretty sure it was entered in the computer. Psychiatry . . . see I did my part, psychiatry consults . . . this was the last time you guys saw me . . . um. . . . .*

MRS. WHEELER: *I never received anything. . . .*

DOCTOR: *The nurse was supposed to schedule you an appointment within one week?*

MR. WHEELER: *Well, they, you haven't been. . . .*

DOCTOR: *It says here a referral, November 20th? So, um. . . .*

MRS. WHEELER: *I did not receive nothing.*

DOCTOR: *They didn't give you an appointment last time when you left?*

MRS. WHEELER: *No.*

DOCTOR: *Okay. You know, what I think may have happened last time. . . .*

MRS. WHEELER: *He is putting me on the antidepressant today. . . .*

DOCTOR: *Okay, terrific. There is one piece of good news that we have had in the past three months.*

MR. WHEELER: *But there's all kind of bad news. The good luck that I have had so far is mine has went into remission!*

DOCTOR: *Terrific.*

Disorder and fragmentation of care, so much a part of the public hospital system, were apparent throughout the first minutes of Mrs. Wheeler's appointment. Very quickly we see that her doctor, despite being patient centered, was unaware of events of the past few weeks. He was not fully up to date on what doctors she was

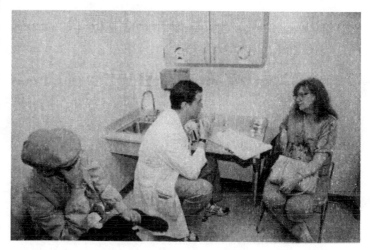

His words say, "I'm in remission." His expression says, "How much more can I take?"

seeing, what tests had been run, or the status of her diagnosis. He was taken aback by her complaint of back pain and reference to disc problems. He was unaware that despite serious psychological issues in her life, she had not been seen by a therapist. In fact, the physician appeared to be on the defensive when he realized that an appointment had not been made:

DOCTOR: *I'm glad you brought up the psychiatry issues. I was wondering if you made it over there. I will try and . . . I mean, so far I did everything I could to get you the appointment.*

MRS. WHEELER: *Uh-huh.*

DOCTOR: *We will try to get you another one.*

MRS. WHEELER: *I have never received nothing, you know. . . . If I would've received something then I would've went, you know.*

I do not mean to imply that this intern was uninterested in Mrs. Wheeler's welfare. To the contrary, he was empathic and patient throughout the appointment. However, he, too, was part of a chaotic and stressed system of care. He would have to answer to his superior if he had made a mistake. His need to figure out his responsibility in the breakdown of care was understandable. In the pecking order of power in the public hospital and teaching medical center, he was vulnerable and overburdened by an extensive caseload. The sad fact was that he would never be able to provide regular, continuous, integrated care to the Wheelers and others like them. The best he could do was to be of service when they came to the clinic, make sound medical decisions, and be empathetic to their sufferings. As we have seen, he did so quite well. In fact, he spent so much time with Mrs. Wheeler that day that it put him significantly behind in his schedule and elicited criticism from staff about "efficient use of time."

DOCTOR: *So we've got a lot of ground to cover today. We have ears, both ears, back, nerves, and the bone pain.*

MR. WHEELER: *And sleepin'.*

MRS. WHEELER: *Sleepin'.*

DOCTOR: *Alright.*

MRS. WHEELER: *I'm still taking his medicine for sleep.*

DOCTOR: *These all yours?*

MRS. WHEELER: *Yes [talking softly, almost inaudible].*

DOCTOR: *Is the pharmacy really shocked when they see this?*

MRS. WHEELER: *All the time.*

DOCTOR: *We went up on this, did we not? On the Buspar? Did that help at all? Nerves are still shot?*

MRS. WHEELER: *Uh-huh.*

DOCTOR: *You have been treated only a while for it or your whole life or just. . . .*

MRS. WHEELER: *For just a short period.*

DOCTOR: *Okay. How recently?*

MRS. WHEELER: *Just during this.*

DOCTOR: *Okay. Is it only now that's when you really needed the medicine?*

MRS. WHEELER: *Uh-huh.*

DOCTOR: *. . . with this diagnosis.*

MRS. WHEELER: *I have, you know, been getting worse with this. . . .*

MR. WHEELER: *Now, her nerves. . . .*

MRS. WHEELER: *My mother ignored me, cussing me out because she is drunk. I can't take her. . . .*

MR. WHEELER: *[interjecting] Mouth.*

DOCTOR: *Her what?*

MRS. WHEELER: *Her mouth.*

DOCTOR: *Her mouth.*

MRS. WHEELER: *She has an abusive mouth.*

DOCTOR: *Why does your wife put up with this?*

MRS. WHEELER: *I am always having to call her and say, "Hi Mom, how ya doin'?" You know, trying to be obedient, trying to, you know, be a daughter to her, you know, but then. . . .*

MR. WHEELER: *When she gets smart, she'll hang up.*

MRS. WHEELER: *If she is drinking or something she will say, "You bitch, you whore, you no good for nothing."*

MR. WHEELER: *And then she'll hang up on her.*

MRS. WHEELER: *When she starts that I get nervous and I just hang up.*

DOCTOR: *That's a terrible situation.*

MRS. WHEELER: *And, you see a lot of fires, right. I have been in a fire. My grandmother's house burnt to the ground. I see these fires today, and it, you know. . . .*

DOCTOR: *Causes you problems?*

MRS. WHEELER: *Causes me problems.*

DOCTOR: *Are there a lot of fires where you live?*

MRS. WHEELER: *We have a lot, there's fires where we live at, there's a lot of fires going on television when we watch TV at night. You see all these fires. . . .*

DOCTOR: *Like on the news?*

The doctor shifted gears in the conversation and picked up an empty bottle of pills that Mrs. Wheeler had brought with her.

DOCTOR: *The amitriptiline . . . Have you been out of this for a while?*

MRS. WHEELER: *Yes.*

DOCTOR: *Did this help with your sleep?*

MRS. WHEELER: *No!*

DOCTOR: *Are you falling asleep and then waking up early or not falling asleep at all?*

MRS. WHEELER: *I'll fall asleep, you know, like I could be watching TV and I'll fall asleep.*

MR. WHEELER: *But when she goes to bed.*

MRS. WHEELER: *. . . and I decide to go to bed and wake up again.*

MR. WHEELER: *And she is wide awake.*

MRS. WHEELER: *I just can't sleep. I've tried everything.*

The conversation returned to a discussion of lymphoma and the diagnostic plan presented by the hematologist. Mrs. Wheeler again expressed fears about her illness, fears about the surgery, and anger at having to wait so long for a biopsy to be performed. The doctor asked, "How can we best help you? You have to let me know as this is a question we will have to work out together." She responded, "Get me well. Get him well." She broke down in tears at this point, and the doctor offered comfort.

DOCTOR: *It's okay, you can cry. Don't be embarrassed because of this. What do you think about most of the time?*

MRS. WHEELER: *Him. I don't know how life can go on. I just wish it would get over with. . . . Everything worries me.*

DOCTOR: *I think you worry a lot to begin with. Your nerves were so jittery even before this.*

MRS. WHEELER: *I been through so much. My mother beat on me when I was growing up.*

MR. WHEELER: *Like I told her, when she starts bitching on the phone, hang up on her . . . and I've got to start hanging up on her.*

DOCTOR: *It's not a good situation.*

MRS. WHEELER: *I try to be her daughter by calling her and seeing how she is. I can't stand when she talks to me on the phone: "I'm alright . . . I'm going to kill myself . . . You don't care about me . . . you bitch . . . you whore."*

DOCTOR: *Has she tried suicide in the past?*

MRS. WHEELER: *Yeah, she's tried suicide.*

DOCTOR: *How many times has she tried suicide?*

MR. WHEELER: *I think she is trying it now because she is drinking herself to death.*

DOCTOR: *But purposefully . . . what has she tried in the past?*

MRS. WHEELER: *She is drinking herself to death. She says she is going to get the gun that they've got and blow her brains out. All this stuff. . . . .*

DOCTOR: *Besides just saying, you know, threats, has she ever tried it?*

MRS. WHEELER: *No. The only thing that I have ever seen her try is taking a bottle of aspirin.*

DOCTOR: *Oh, she did?*

MRS. WHEELER: *. . . and it didn't phase her.*

DOCTOR: *Does that still happen, are you still abused at all?*

MRS. WHEELER: *She don't hit me now, but she used to when I worked with her, she used to hit me.*

DOCTOR: *Does anybody hit you?*

MRS. WHEELER: *No, not now. If she comes over, she is not allowed to touch me.*

MR. WHEELER: *Because that's when I jump in.*

DOCTOR: *Superman!*

As one can readily see, an awful lot is going on. Their illness experiences were having a dismantling effect. Mrs. Wheeler was experiencing severe emotional disturbance that was setting the stage for her eventual emotional breakdown. She worried continuously about coming apart, likening her "crumbling back" to her "crumbling life." She lived in terror and experienced irrational fears, most notably of fire and of medical procedures. She perseverated about widowhood and how she would not be able to live without her husband. Most of all she was haunted by a fear that Mr. Wheeler would die in his sleep and that she would wake up in the morning next to her dead husband. "I cannot deal with that," she would say, sometimes in front of him.

Additionally, Judy was in an unhealthy and abusive relationship with her mother. She was unable to sever the dysfunctional tie to her mother and begin to heal the poisonous effects of their relationship. In many ways illness had become the imprimatur of Mrs. Wheeler's life. She defined much of herself in terms of symptoms and equated her life to disease, ailments, and associated sufferings. Her life was equally defined by her husband's illness and worries about their future. Thus, in innumerable ways she was becoming emotionally and psychologically imprisoned in a world that was relentlessly beating her down and from which she found little reprieve.

In a different form, Mr. Wheeler was also in a state of emotional decline. His main response throughout was a mixture of anger and stoicism. In the nine months I knew him, I saw him smile only four times, one of which was during the miscommunication debacle in the oncology clinic. He would occasionally kid around and was always glad to see me, yet a continual sense of despair weighed heavily on him. He dwelled on both his disease and his anger about being a patient in County Hospital. His primary source of refuge from anger was his television. He leased a fifty-five-inch TV from one of the local rental centers, which flourish particularly in poor inner-city neighborhoods. The TV was disproportionately large for the room it was in, and it truly was the focal point of many of their days. As husband and wife, they sequestered themselves in front of the television. There, they took their phone calls, received the occasional visitor, and ate all their meals. In their seemingly desperate search for meaning, they began tuning in to religious programming. Whether it

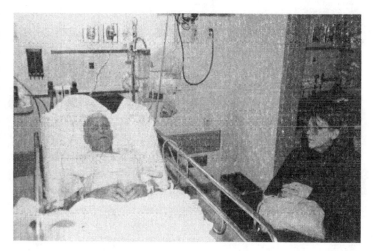

Persistently bitter about being a patient in the public hospital, Mr. Wheeler remained dependent on its services, no matter how begrudgingly. He is shown here one hour after arrival in the ER.

was television evangelism or network shows such as *Touched by an Angel*, Mr. Wheeler looked to these programs as he searched for answers and comfort during this difficult time.

One Saturday afternoon Mr. Wheeler became increasingly lightheaded and was having difficulty breathing. He and his wife engaged in an argument about going to the hospital. She wanted to call an ambulance, but he fought with her about it. Being so angry at County, he wanted nothing to do with going there. They spent the rest of the day arguing, she trying to persuade him to go, him resisting. Finally, at 6:00 AM on Sunday at her wit's end, Mrs. Wheeler called me at home, and I strongly advised her to call 911. When Mr. Wheeler was informed that I would meet them at the hospital, his resistance ended, and he agreed to go. Feeling reassured that someone they trusted would be there as an advocate enabled him to temporarily put aside his anger and mistrust. Mrs. Wheeler called for an ambulance, and Mr. Wheeler was taken to the emergency room, where a cardiac assessment was begun. Interestingly, none of the anger that prevented him from calling 911 sooner could be seen in his interaction with the staff. In fact, despite his brooding, he was compliant, quiet, and unobtrusive for the nine hours he was in the ER. As already mentioned, like many indigent patients Mr. Wheeler tended to internalize rather than express his anger. He never felt adequately empowered to verbalize his discontent, civilly or otherwise. Thus, he would acquiesce in "perturbed acceptance" to his care and caregivers, resentfully grumbling to himself.

The preliminary work-up in the ER indicated that Mr. Wheeler had suffered a heart attack. Midday on Sunday he was admitted to the intensive care unit (ICU). There, his anger heightened, and doubt about his "remission" began to sink in. In the midst of all that was happening, he began to think about dying and intensified his search for God in hope of finding some explanation for his sufferings.

This particular deepening of anger was fueled directly by past experience. The ICU elicited strong negative memories for both him and Judy. They both strongly felt he had received disrespectful and discourteous treatment during a previous stay. They brought strong negative emotions from the prior admission to the current one. His complaints ranged from the food being inedible to not being able to get a blanket or pillow to the attitude of a particular nurse. Mr. Wheeler recounted:

> I asked for a gown and a blanket for that Friday and didn't get it until Sunday. And one smart-aleck nurse. Boy, I mean she was a downright smartalec. There was no pleasin' that woman. When it come to food time, you know the way you cook spaghetti and drain it and then it turns hard on ya, kind of a brownish color, like that lamp shade, well that's what it looked like, with sauce poured on it. I told 'em I ain't eatin' that shit. So, Monday morning came and I told the doctors to check my ass out of there.

Unable to get a blanket and gown for two days and not able to get a different pillow intensified his anger and mistrust. "I was so damn mad that I wanted to come home Saturday," he said. Judy added, "He was raising all kind of trouble with me because I was the one who put him in the hospital to begin with." She then proceeded to explain why she finally called 911 despite their mutual anger at County. "But after taking two nitroglycerines, it didn't work. There was only one thing to do. I had to call the ambulance." He responded, "I know it, but when you get treated that way you don't want to . . . hell, you want to get out of here." Things had deteriorated to the point, in Mr. Wheeler's perspective, that when he was asked to provide an overall assessment of the care he previously received in the ICU, he wrathfully said, "Piss poor!"

Beyond problems with the food and getting a blanket, gown, and pillow, there was the continuing disrespectful and noncompassionate attitude of the nurse in charge of his care. "Her attitude, based on a scale of 1 to 10, take 10 as the worst, it would have to be a 10," he said. "She was just rude. Everything she said, there was something rude about it." After a pause in which the anger he was feeling was apparent on his face, he resumed: "She was a bitch. . . . Hateful! Towards everybody."

Undoubtedly, the sources of anger in Mr. Wheeler were diverse and pervasive. He was "pissed off" at being sick. Despite all the talk about remission, deep down he was worried about dying. His finances were a mess (remember that he lived in the dark most of the time), he felt that he had been misdiagnosed, and his wife had recently learned that she had lymphoma. Furthermore, he was suffering all this in significant isolation from family and community support. In short, physically he felt awful most of the time, personally he was steeped in anger, and socially he felt the sting of loneliness and isolation. Part of the reason his anger was surging at this point was that denial—his belief that he was in remission—was increasingly difficult to sustain. Recognizing that he was getting sicker, not better, he was becoming increasingly resentful and full of rage. They both felt that the staff at County, especially in the ICU, did not understand or relate to their sufferings. Consequently, both Bill and Judy saw them as cold, indifferent, and rude.

The quibbling that occurred regarding whether he would go the hospital needs to be understood in light of these memories and perceptions. Mr. Wheeler further explained:

> I wanted no part of that kind of treatment. None! Have you ever been through that kind of deal? When you get treated like that you get gun shy, and I got gun shy . . . and it's not the first time I've been mistreated.

In order to grasp what was going on in the life of Mr. Wheeler at this point, it is important to understand that his indignation was rising as his capacity to maintain self-deceit and delusion was waning. As part of confronting the new realities of his illness, his belief in remission was being directly challenged, as was Judy's. She began:

MRS. WHEELER: *We don't know how long he's going to live.*

MR. WHEELER: *Well, they told me it was in remission, and with me staying sick constantly, I don't think it was ever in remission.*

He went on to state that he felt his doctors were lying to him, but his wife had a slightly different take. "I think he was just trying to play a guessing game because they can't find no lymph nodes in his neck . . . but that doesn't mean that it is in remission. The way he is doing, he's not in remission." Mr. Wheeler, now forced into the difficult process of adjusting his view of the illness, implicitly concurred. "And, I'll throw up for days at a time." Thus, for the first time he was letting his wife know that he was beginning to believe that his so-called remission was an illusion. Irritated, he concluded, "Well, I'm going to talk to him and point-blank ask him how much longer I've got." Mrs. Wheeler, who had never before expressed her suspicions to Bill that he was not in remission, worried that he might not make it to his next oncology appointment. Directly in front of her husband, she said,

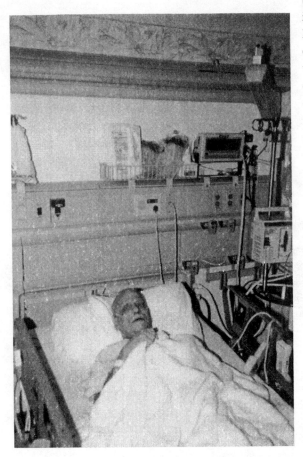

As his belief in remission fades, a resentful and angry Mr. Wheeler searches for God in the intensive care unit.

I worry that he will just not live until February 3rd . . . That's why I'm not sleeping. I think I am up every hour on the hour just to see if he is breathing or not. And that right there shows me it's still not in remission. And it's scaring me to even think about me going through the same thing myself.

There were many difficult things going on in the life of the Wheelers. Throughout the swiftly progressing course of events over the previous six weeks, the quality of their lives had been significantly diminished, and their faith in the future had been shattered. They faced not only the severity of his illness, but the disillusionment that was emerging from the crack in their mutual masquerade about remission. Mrs. Wheeler again voiced her fears. "He seems to be getting worse," to which Mr. Wheeler added, "I think it's still there because my belly hurts constantly." His wife, reaffirming the extent of his pain, added, "It don't let up." It was as if a catharsis of sorts was taking place. Mr. Wheeler, going further and admitting for the first time that he was "terminally ill and won't get well," offered the following explanation:

> Well, that's the way I understand it. Because you wouldn't be this way if you was in remission . . . if you was in remission you wouldn't be as sick as I've been.

On their own, without the benefit of an open conversation with physicians, they were coming to a painful realization of how sick he really was. As they discussed the seriousness of his condition, there seemed to be a perceptible urgency to have this discussion, as if they had come to a point at which they could finally talk about their private fears. It was in this new framework of understanding that Mr. Wheeler began actively to think about dying. In doing so he intensified his search for meaning and spiritual comfort, a process that led him to reflect about his wife, God, and the purpose of life.

As already indicated, Mr. and Mrs. Wheeler were rediscovering their love for each other. In the face of the belligerence of disease, they were carving out a personalized form of dignity in their dependency on each other. Mr. Wheeler put his suffering into perspective. "Death won't be so bad. No pain. You never have to worry about any pain and you don't have to worry about your gas bills, your light bills, anything like that. What's going to hurt me is just leaving my wife. I could spend the next 100 years with her." With these simple words he was expressing, perhaps unwittingly, several important insights:

- Life's meaning is found in family and relationships.
- The physical agony of disease would be relieved upon death.
- The everyday harm and injury inflicted on his life by poverty would end when he died.

During this time Mr. Wheeler worried about Judy. He was concerned not just about her battle with lymphoma but about how she would cope with his death. In the ICU he lay in his bed praying that she would have the strength to endure his death and survive without him:

> I talk to Him (God) about her all the time. I pray to God to help her, to guide her. Give her strength; a funeral is not for the dead person. It's for the person that's alive.

It was only over the past month or so that Mr. Wheeler had begun praying and thinking about God. In fact, he had been "thinking about God quite a bit lately and wondering what the big picture is about." When I had first met him eight months earlier, he told me that he was not religious and was not at all sure that there was a God. His recent sufferings had brought God into his life, and a relationship of sorts began to develop. Ironically, Mr. Wheeler was not trying to reach out to God in order to strike a bargain and effect a cure. He was not even asking God to control his pain and relieve his suffering. All he wanted was, "Just His love. Just His love. That means a whole lot. It means that you are forgiven for all the sins that you've done, and He forgives you for them." In the ICU at the public hospital surrounded by a sophisticated array of life-prolonging technology, Mr. Wheeler was talking to God and beginning to feel his presence. "You know, they say there is no God, but there has to be a God on account of the good things that did happen to you in life. They say that's in your spiritual mind, about having a God. It must be in my spiritual mind, but there is a God." When asked how he recognized God's presence, he replied simply, "It's a gut feeling. God is here in this room with me."

Mr. Wheeler was both hopeful and regretful at this point. He was hopeful that God's love would comfort him and see him through these, his darkest days. On the other hand he was regretful and felt some pangs of conscience that God was not a part of his life before now, especially during all his years of "drinking and running around." It would seem that Mr. Wheeler was putting forth another important insight that emerged from his sufferings: Faith and belief in God can nourish the human spirit during good and bad times, perhaps as no other human enterprise can.

After about a week in the ICU, Mr. Wheeler began to look and feel better. He regained some strength and was told that he would be able to go home in a few days. He became more hopeful, and he once again began to think that he might be able to beat this thing.

> Like last Friday and Saturday, I didn't think I was going to make it. Now I do . . . I'm fightin' more today than I had all day Saturday, like you know when you say you're not going to give up on something? That's the way I feel. I'm not going to give up. I'm not. I'm going to fight it every step of the way.

Reflecting on his new optimism, Mr. Wheeler admitted that it was hard to know exactly what the future would be, but in the very next breath he said,

> I know I'm going to live long enough to see her get old with me.

Mr. Wheeler was doing better and had been stabilized. He had incurred some heart damage. It was also discovered that he had recently suffered a mild stroke, but thanks to the skill of his doctors death had been forestalled. He might still die at any time, but he was well enough to be released, so he went home, somewhat grateful for the life-saving care he had received. Even so, he was still angry and resentful about being sick and being a patient in County Hospital. In fact, the day he was released he told his wife, "If I have to go back to the hospital tell them to send me to another hospital." Of course, however, being a patient in County's indigent program, Mr. Wheeler had no choice but to go there for his health care.

The hope and spirit of optimism that was briefly resurrected toward the end of his stay in the ICU quickly faded after he returned home. He was growing weaker. He had trouble getting up and walking, his stomach hurt constantly, and he would throw up whenever he ate solid food. Overall, as his disease progressed worry and anger seized even greater control of his life. They seemed to become his most intimate companions. He continued to watch religious programming in his search for meaning and comfort. The sad fact, however, was that Mr. Wheeler's search for God was precipitated by necessity and desperation. Unlike J. W., Mrs. Angel, and Annie, whose faith was a significant and continuous part of who they were throughout their lives, his relationship with God lacked discipline, commitment, and history. Born out of the urgency of despair, his faith was fragile. Therefore, it could not stem the tidal wave of suffering he was facing. He recognized this, but still he struggled to believe. "There must be a God. They wouldn't put it on television if it weren't true," he stated. Upon being asked what message he would like to offer other people by which he would be remembered, he quickly and simply said:

Keep an eye on your health, have it checked more frequently, and put yourself in God's hands.

He went on to say that he wished he had done both more faithfully throughout his life. He seemed haunted by a sense of social and spiritual isolation. The resulting emptiness fueled a growing feeling of hopelessness, especially as hope for a cure faded. His search for God's love was never fully realized. Nonetheless, he continued to yearn for spiritual connection and comfort, but this yearning took place entirely in isolation. He never attended church, nor did he receive a pastoral visit or participate in any religious rituals during this time. Thus, without the spiritual support of others and lacking an authentic connection to an established religious tradition, his longing for spiritual comfort remained unfulfilled.

Communal support was similarly infrequent throughout his illness. Former coworkers never visited, Mrs. Wheeler's son visited three times in nine months, his sisters never visited, his brother visited once, and friends and neighbors were seldom part of their daily lives. Their main source of connection to the world and distraction from suffering continued to be the television. In this framework, the fragility of his faith coupled with extensive social isolation deepened his anguish. Hour after hour, day after day, week after week, he would lie on the couch or sit in a chair in desolation and gloom.

Not only was this a time of dejection for Mr. Wheeler, it was a personally difficult time for me as well. I was witnessing his physical decline with great sorrow,

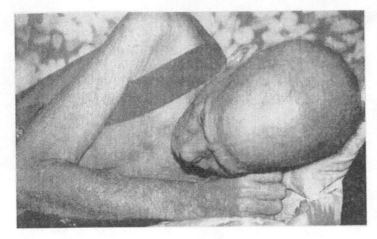

Becoming increasingly spiritless and hopeless.

wondering why he had not been referred to hospice. Some of the services offered by hospice, it seemed, would have been welcomed sources of support for both of them. Mr. Wheeler was determined to come to grips with the remission issue and once more remarked that, "Next time I see him I am going to ask him point-blank how long I have." Because the appointment to which he was referring was sixteen days away, I worried that in the interim unnecessary suffering would transpire. After consulting with colleagues, I made the decision to explain hospice to him and see whether he might be interested. Despite the fact that I knew I was now starting to interfere with the process of his care, I felt a moral duty to have the conversation.

I went to his house one Friday morning shortly after his discharge from the ICU. I began by asking if they had ever heard of hospice, and they responded, "No." I briefly offered an explanation of its philosophy and services and asked if they would like to hear more. "Yes, I would," Mr. Wheeler replied. So I continued, and the conversation flowed easily. They both indicated that they would like to have a nurse come by to explain the program further. Anxious to move quickly, Dr. G arranged for the hospice nurse to

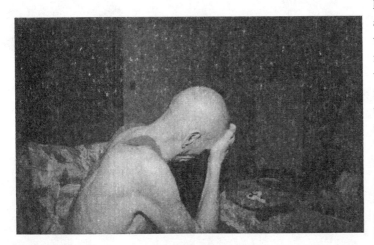

Pondering the reasons for his suffering, Mr. Wheeler was never able to reach a comforting or meaningful explanation.

come by that afternoon. She spent an hour and a half explaining the philosophy of hospice, what it meant, and what it could offer. This interaction was a point of enormous reckoning for Mr. Wheeler, who listened intently to every word she spoke. He was mostly quiet throughout the conversation, changing positions on the couch frequently. He vomited twice during the talk and appeared to be in deep, somber thought from beginning to end. He expressed keen interest in the program, as did Judy.

However, when the nurse asked if he would like to enroll, he firmly said, "No." Gently probing for his reasons, the hospice nurse asked him why. All that Mr. Wheeler would offer is that he needed to hear from his oncologist that the chemotherapy was not working, and he wanted to hear it, "Point-blank and outright." He made this point emphatically on several occasions during the week that followed, demonstrating an important lesson, namely, that the words and authority of medical specialists carry a distinct power upon which

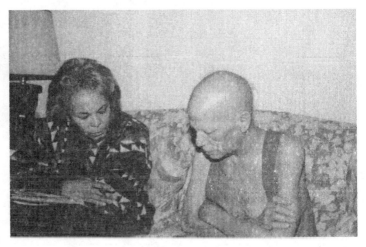

Hospice talk begins.

vulnerable patients are strongly reliant. In order to make the transition from curative to palliative treatment, Mr. Wheeler needed the approval of his oncologist. Although it is regrettable that he struggled with the "misbelief" that he was in remission during the preceding five months, it seemed only fitting that the individual who gave him this hope should be the one to formally dismantle it. Thus, hospice would have to wait.

Despite declining the services of hospice, Mr. Wheeler was coming to understand that he was getting close to death. He expressed his desire to die at home and to be cremated thereafter. He had been having conversations with his wife about staying home to die. She insisted that she could not cope with that and told him on many occasions that she was terrified of waking up one morning to find him dead in bed next to her. Privately Mr. Wheeler assured me, "Don't worry, just you wait and see. She's a tough old gal, you know." Mr. Wheeler was confident that she would have the strength to endure his dying at home, and he was right in a way. These conversations with Judy, in part prompted by the hospice discussion, were part of a developing awareness that he was not in remission, and that that pretense could no longer be maintained. In fact, with increasing candor they both spoke about the gravity of his situation:

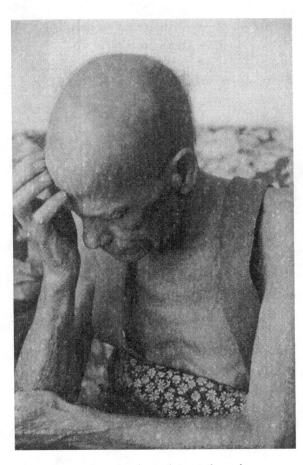

The understanding that he is dying is brought to a new level.

MRS. WHEELER: *They say don't let his heart rate go over ninety, because of the bottom of his heart being dead. They said he can have another heart attack in just a second.*

MR. WHEELER: *And if it was in remission I wouldn't be getting sick at my stomach like this.*

MRS. WHEELER: *And he had to have blood while he was in the hospital. He needed blood . . . he probably still needs more, and that's due to the fact of the cancer.*

DAVID: *Did you ever believe he was in remission?*

MRS. WHEELER: *No, not to my knowledge. I wouldn't call it remission.*

DAVID: *You said that privately to me quite a while ago that you weren't sure. Did you ever tell that to Mr. Wheeler?*

MRS. WHEELER: *No. I wanted him to be happy instead of worrying, you know?*

MR. WHEELER: *And to have the hope?*

MRS. WHEELER: *I try to keep the hope.*

MR. WHEELER: *Well, the hope's gone on account of the way I've been sick.*

MRS. WHEELER: *And the hope I've got is gone.*

DAVID: *For him?*

MRS. WHEELER: *Uh-huh . . . and for myself.*

DAVID: *For yourself too?*

MR. WHEELER: *Like right now, I'm feeling like I'm going to throw up.*

MRS. WHEELER: *There's nothing he can eat. There's nothing keeping his food down. He keeps throwing it back up. He hasn't had a thing to eat today. There ain't nothing nobody can do, except watch him.*

DAVID: *Is that hard for you?*

MRS. WHEELER: *Very hard.*

DAVID: *Do you feel like he is dying before your eyes?*

MRS. WHEELER: *Uh-huh. That's why I can't sleep. I was getting the treatments for, you know, psychiatric treatments . . . but since he was in the hospital I haven't been able to go to the psychiatrist. I'm supposed to be going over here to see this psychiatrist over here at Peoples [a community health center that is part of CHS]. I haven't been able to go. I don't want to leave him alone. I try to get him . . . he's not even driving the truck anymore. We're letting a neighbor drive it, and they're not trying to do nothing for me either. You know, they said they was going to operate . . . but they didn't. They said there's no reason to. The only thing that can do anything would be chemotherapy, and seeing what he is going through, I don't want it.*

It is important to remember that throughout her husband's tribulations, Mrs. Wheeler was coping with her own illness. While witnessing the decline of her husband, she was fearful of following a similar course of decline. She began to debate whether to opt for chemotherapy after watching what her husband had endured. Despite being concerned about her illness, most of her focus was on her husband's torment and her associated fear of his death. Additionally, caring for him with minimal help for months had taken its toll. She was weary, and Bill was exhausted. Moreover, the emotional drain on her was nerve-racking. She spent most of her time worried and tense, as if she were sitting on the edge of a cliff and waiting for an axe to fall. Her husband, knowing how fragile she was, strove to protect her by keeping things from her. Smart in her own way and largely in tune with him, she knew that he often pretended he felt better than he actually did. Unfortunately, his pretense mostly seemed to increase her stress and worry:

> He's afraid to tell me he's in a lot of pain because it'll worry me. It's like I'm getting ready to go off on a nervous breakdown. I just wish I knew a little bit more about being a nurse. You know, knowing what to do. I don't like to call the hospital all the time. In situations like this, I don't know what to do . . . and that's hurtin' me. Then they try to tell me to keep my nerves down. How am I going to do that?

One got the impression that seeing her husband day in and day out steeped in sickness, suffering, and despondency was bringing her to the brink of collapse. Despite being a "tough old gal," she appeared to be nearing her breaking point. Her back pain was worsening, and she periodically used a walker to get around the house.

Her dizziness was being aggravated by the stress, as was the ringing in her ears. There was virtually no joy in her life and precious little comfort. Her visage revealed an inner anguish, as did her words:

> You know, to live with somebody like this and to see what's going on with him, it's too hard. And, all alone. I could scream and nobody's going to hear me. You know what I'm saying, don't you? The next door neighbor is always gone, and there is nobody else to hear or to help me.

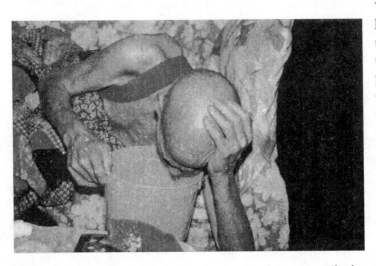

Despite being so sick and truly knowing he was dying, Mr. Wheeler chose not to enroll in hospice.

Mr. and Mrs. Wheeler were in a holding pattern at this point, and, as their words emphasize, their social isolation was acute. Not being enrolled in hospice yet knowing that he was not going to get well put them both in a state of medical limbo and uncertainty. Be this as it may, they had chosen to wait until the oncology clinic appointment to "clear the air and get the facts as they are." As it turned out, they did not have to wait the entire sixteen-day period for this to happen. Mr. Wheeler was having acute stomach pain and difficulty breathing. Too sick to argue against calling 911, he was rushed to the ER and was directly admitted to the hospital. In the fragmented and overburdened schedule at County Hospital, his oncologist staffed the clinic only once a week for half a day. Knowing that Dr. Lens would be on campus Wednesday morning, Mr. Wheeler put in a request to see him. The doctor visited him in the hospital after finishing clinic, and Mr. Wheeler asked him directly about his progress. He was told, "We never expected you to live this long, and for patients with your type of tumor who live as long as you have, the average survival is two to five years." This incensed Mr. Wheeler, who said shortly afterward, "See, he's lying again!" He continued, "They should have told me the whole truth in the first place." Resentful over the way his hope had been agonizingly crushed over the past months, he realized that the initial hopefulness engendered by the "remission talk" that day in oncology was ultimately a disservice. While at first bringing a rare smile to his face ("You'll remember I was grinning from ear to ear," he reminded me), it intensified his suffering by creating unrealistic expectations. Privately in the hallway later on, Mrs. Wheeler expressed a similar sentiment and anger when she said, "They really did lie because you and me both know it was never in remission." Bill expressed his displeasure, saying if he could freely speak to his doctors, he would tell them that above anything else.

Why did you lie? Why didn't you tell me the truth from the get-go like I asked?

In the complicated institutional organization of the public hospital, however, where lack of integration and continuity of care are a problem, it turned out that the doctor who assumed his oncological care was different from the one who delivered the bad news to him in the first place. Thus, although he was correct in noting that he requested full disclosure, as "honesty is the best policy," he never made that wish known to any of the oncologists who subsequently took care of him, nor did they ask him how much he wished to know. Always prone to internalize his discontent, Mr. Wheeler never expressed his anger or told the doctor directly of his dissatisfaction. Instead, he broached the topic of hospice with Dr. Lens, and the remainder of the visit revolved around a discussion of the appropriateness and benefits of hospice care. Mr. Wheeler, having finally received referral and "approval" from the specialist upon whom he was so dependent and with whom he was so angry, was now ready to enroll in hospice. The arrangements were made before he was discharged from what would turn out to be his final visit to County Hospital.

Upon arriving home Mr. Wheeler continued to complain about County. "I am just a number to them, ya know. If I had any choice I'd go to any other hospital but that one." In some ways Mr. Wheeler's complaints were legitimate. As discussed in Chapter 3, clinic care is chaotic, fragmented, and full of long waits. In the hospital an ever changing coterie of interns and residents make care seem very impersonal. Immense errors in communication occurred between him and the oncologists. He did receive detestable treatment in the ICU. Although those regrettable incidents in the ICU were mitigated by the fact that they occurred over the weekend of a major snowstorm and cold spell that created a shortage of both staff and blankets, this explanation was of little comfort to him. There can be little doubt that he was diagnosed late in his illness because he was an indigent patient who relied so much on the ER for his health care. Consequently, his anger and discontent had basis. Also, all Mr. Wheeler knew was that he requested to be told the truth from the beginning. He had asked the doctor in the hospital who told him of the diagnosis to "let me know all the facts as they are." In the final analysis, however, that never happened, and he suffered the disservice of false hope and shattered expectations.

Inasmuch as resentment and indignation became a kind of trademark for Mr. Wheeler, they can also be understood as a way of coping and a means of feeling empowered. When much of his personhood was being brutally demolished by disease, he took a refuge of sorts in his ability to complain. In grumbling, griping, and making a fuss, even if only indirectly expressed, he was maintaining some control and asserting a capacity to act while so much was being taken away. It is not pressing too far to suggest that Mr. Wheeler needed his anger and became dependent on it in order to maintain some form of empowerment in his life.

Another interesting means of empowerment for him was eating foods that he was not supposed to eat. Up until two weeks before his death, he was still eating spicy chicken wings that Judy would make for him. Despite having been told he should avoid spicy food and be on a clear liquid diet with, perhaps, some pudding or Jell-O, Mr. Wheeler did not care. "I'll have 'em again," he asserted, "whenever I want." When I asked why he had been eating the wings when he knew he would get sick, he curtly responded, "Because I wanted 'em." When pushed a little further to explain his choice to do something that would only increase his physical suffering, he said,

Because I'm still running my life.

Spicy chicken wings, like his anger and discontent, were forms of self-assertion. He resented being told that he could not eat certain foods at a time when so much else was being lost.

MR. WHEELER: *If I was in the hospital and they told me I couldn't have it, I'll betcha I'd have it. Because she'd bring it to me. I was in there one time. Monday, wasn't it?*

MRS. WHEELER: *Yeah.*

MR. WHEELER: *They told me I couldn't have a hamburger and a shake.*

MRS. WHEELER: *I didn't know that.*

MR. WHEELER: *But I wanted a hamburger and shake.*

MRS. WHEELER: *I didn't know it.*

MR. WHEELER: *Guess what I had?*

DAVID: *A hamburger and shake?*

MR. WHEELER: *A hamburger and a shake.*

DAVID: *Did you go get it for him?*

MRS. WHEELER: *He called me and told me he wanted a hamburger and a shake and I went and got it for him.*

In a very complicated way, sometimes things that may not be clinically beneficial for the body may be good or necessary for the patient as a person. Furthermore, those in the "dying well–happy death movement" who reject anger as "an immature stage" in the dying process, most notably Kübler-Ross and her followers, may be imposing an unrealistic standard on dying persons. Some patients, such as Mr. Wheeler, need to be difficult. In fact, typically he became most animated when complaining.   He seemed to get energy by constantly criticizing the care he received. In all honesty, given the realities of his indigent life as a cancer patient, his anger is understandable. In a paradoxical way, it was even beneficial and energizing for him. Anger was one of Mr. Wheeler's coping mechanisms.

The end of Mr. Wheeler's life was approaching. Hospice had been involved for a few

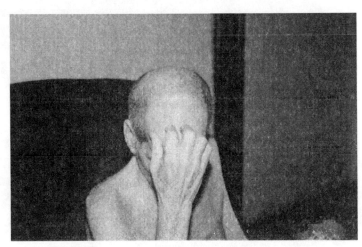

When asked about what he is thinking these days, a despondent Mr. Wheeler responded, "Not much."

weeks with mixed results. The nurse was helpful in talking about advanced directives and facilitating further discussion about funeral arrangements. She was very responsive to all their calls as his symptoms worsened and quickly became a trusted and valuable caretaker. Mrs. Wheeler was especially grateful for the tips she was given on how to care for him. She particularly appreciated being taught symptoms and signs to watch for as he got closer to death. On the other hand, hospice did little to ease their social and spiritual isolation. No volunteers visited, and the chaplain came only twice and disappeared from their lives thereafter. As Mrs. Wheeler stated, "The chaplain didn't come this week. He wasn't here last week either. I don't know what's wrong unless he's sick or busy or something. I'm being a tough old gal now."

The search for God and meaning continued in its usual form for the Wheelers. As she disclosed,

> I am getting through this by asking for God's help. I felt his presence here last night. Yes. I was watching channel 40 [religious programming] all night long, and that was comforting.

Dependable social and spiritual support would have been welcome at any time but was particularly needed at this point, given the depths of their isolation and suffering. This was a painful period for not only the obvious reasons. An unexpected source of upheaval had made its way into their lives. Somehow, a former sister-in-law, the sister of Bill's estranged wife thirty years ago, discovered he was dying and passed that information on to someone who showed up on their doorstep two weeks before his death. This person was his son—a son he had never met nor even knew that he had. As the story unfolded, it was revealed that his former wife had become pregnant just prior to their bitter separation and never let him know. When this thirty-year-old man, along with his fiancé, rang the doorbell and introduced himself, it brought unforeseen confusion into the Wheeler household. The son and his fiancé sat in chairs next to Mr. Wheeler, who was now in a wheelchair. They were quiet, as this was a difficult situation for them as well. Mrs. Wheeler, despite being unnerved by their arrival, tried to ease the tension and offered her support to this stranger and newfound stepson.

MRS. WHEELER: *(speaking to David) It's kind of tough for him. He is just now learning that this is his father, and they have been separated for a long time.*

SON: *I knew he was my father, but we have been apart for thirty years.*

MRS. WHEELER: *Yeah, today was the first time he had seen him. And it's pretty rough on him, but I think he can handle it. If I can handle it, you can handle it.*

SON: *Yeah.*

DAVID: *(speaking to Bill) Are you glad to see him?*

MR. WHEELER: *(in a state of confusion) Nope. Uh-uh (no).*

The visit lasted about three hours, during which Mr. Wheeler would nod off to sleep and experience some episodes of confusion. Despite the awkwardness of the encounter, which included conflicting memories and accounts of what had occurred in the past, they all did remarkably well by one another. The son felt reassured by Mrs. Wheeler's overtures of acceptance. He also was aware that there would not be much time in the future to see the father he had never known. However, he tried to make the best of a difficult situation. Mostly, the conversation dealt with what had been happening medically and what was happening at the moment. At the end of their visit, everyone hugged. Mr. Wheeler stated, "The pity is that this is the first time in thirty years I have seen my son . . . but that's also a good thing. I wished I had seen him sooner, but I couldn't." Thus, before dying Mr. Wheeler would have to endure more regret, namely, the shame, sorrow, and remorse of learning about a son he never even knew he had. In a moment of soul searching brought on by this visit, he said, "I should have done a lot of things differently thirty years ago." He then went on to offer two additional lessons to be delivered to those who would read about his experiences:

• Don't let nobody else run your life.
• Put somebody that loves you in your life.

Shortly thereafter, at 1:00 on a Saturday afternoon, Bill Wheeler died. Cared for by Judy, he died at home in bed. Although the days preceding his death exhausted her, in a strange way it was a good time for them. He fully submitted to her care, and she took great pride in being able to see him into his

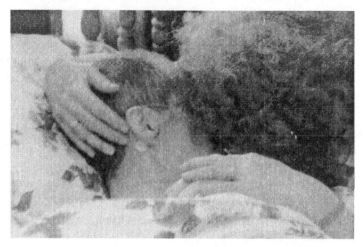

His request to die at home was fulfilled.

death, thereby honoring his wish to die at home. After he died she lovingly touched him, knelt by his side, cried, kissed him, stroked his head, and fondled his hands, aligning his wedding ring with hers as their hands joined.

Although this was a time of enormous anguish for her, there also was a perceptible sense of relief. She had stated often during the past week, "I'm scared," and "I don't know how much more of this I can take." Along with feeling an overwhelming sense of stress, Judy had exhausted herself by single-handedly caring for Bill around the clock. In fact, she was so worn out that she crawled into bed with him and fell asleep for forty-five minutes next to his cooling body.

Mr. Wheeler's body remained in the bed for about two hours. The

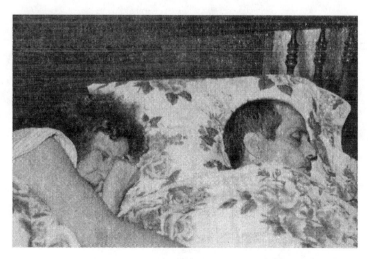

A weary wife sleeps with her husband for the final time.

funeral home had been called immediately after the death, but it took that long for the representatives to arrive. The mortician never said one word to Mrs. Wheeler, business related or otherwise. By the time he arrived she had awakened and was sitting on the couch. Unfortunately, a real opportunity to offer condolence and provide a bit of comfort was missed. It would have taken no more than thirty seconds to say something like, "I am sorry for your loss. Please be assured that we will take very good care of him." Instead, ignoring her completely, he and his assistant proceeded directly to the bedroom and began the ritual of undressing, wrapping, bagging, and moving the body onto a stretcher. They then proceeded straight down the hallway and out of the house without a single word or gesture to Mrs. Wheeler. It is essential to note that Mr. Wheeler did not have money for the funeral, and there was no insurance policy to help cover expenses. His brother, a truck driver who lived in Tennessee, was paying for the viewing and cremation. The services were held at a discount funeral home that almost always arranged low-cost, bottom-of-the-line funerals. I wonder if Mrs. Wheeler, like Mrs. White and many other indigent patients, would have been treated so indifferently had she been able to afford a more expensive funeral or even had been able to pay for the one that had been preplanned by her brother-in-law.

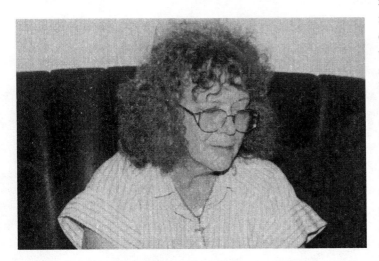

Sadness, severity, and loss acutely line the face of Mrs. Wheeler.

Being unable to pay for the funeral was a source of humiliation, yet it was an important event for her. She was grateful for the help of her brother-in-law, and she insisted on paying for the spray of flowers that covered the casket. She had her hair done and bought a new dress, shoes, and pocketbook, putting all these purchases on the only credit card she possessed.

Afterward, she realized her spending spree was a mistake. Her financial situation had gone from bad to worse, and she did not have the money to pay the credit card bill. A month later the large-screen TV they had leased was repossessed. Nonetheless, for the short term these indulgences helped her go to the wake with her dignity intact, and she was able to get through the viewing and brief service without incident.

Thereafter, she went home alone, and her husband's body was sent to the crematory.

Death brought an end to suffering for Mr. Wheeler, but for Mrs. Wheeler the end of his life was the beginning of a new phase of suffering. Isolated and alone as a widow, she was fearful of beginning the chemotherapy that Mr. Wheeler had convinced her to "give a try." As a result, her anxiety and psychiatric problems deepened. Within a matter of weeks, she entered into a relationship with a previous husband. Judy remarried about a month after Bill died. Although any objective observer would be correct in noting that rushing into another relationship was unhealthy, she was deeply afraid of being alone and desperately needed someone. Tragically, her decision seemed to make sense when viewed within the context of her life, especially its suffering and isolation.

Remarrying did not end her suffering. Judy got involved with a fringe, fanatic religious group. She experienced delusions. She complained that ghosts were invading her bedroom and haunting her throughout the night. She believed that she was going to be able to sue Mr. Wheeler's former employer for wrongful death. He had repaired car radiators at a garage, and she was convinced that his cancer was the result of job-related mercury poisoning. When asked about this, she relayed that a prominent attorney was taking the case and that they had expert medical testimony to support it. When asked about the medical expert, she replied that the doctor was "the

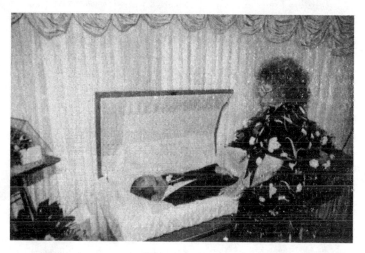

Final farewell.

big cheese." Very quickly Mrs. Wheeler was losing touch with reality and was on the threshold of a nervous breakdown. The absence of continuous medical and psychiatric care, along with the lack of social support, helped to set the stage for this breakdown. When it happened, it came violently.

One Saturday night six weeks after Mr. Wheeler died, Mrs. Wheeler was having extreme delusions about ghosts haunting her. She believed Bill's ghost was following her around and breathing a cool breath on her neck and shoulders. Terrified, she came apart, trashing her house and screaming at the top of her lungs. She smashed lamps, threw furniture, broke a television, and smashed the urn containing Mr. Wheeler's ashes, scattering them all over the place. The disturbance was so boisterous that neighbors called the police. Upon their arrival an ambulance was called, and with a police escort Mrs. Wheeler was immediately taken to the ER. She was assessed, sedated, and admitted to the in-patient psychiatric unit at County Hospital.

It would seem that Mr. Wheeler was correct only in part. She was "a tough old gal" and was able to accompany him into his death and allow him to die at home. What he did not realize while consumed by his own ordeal, however, was the depth of her fragility and vulnerability. Consequently, he was unable to anticipate that her accumulated sufferings were destined to push her over the top emotionally and psychologically.

Their tribulations in the final year of Mr. Wheeler's life were severe. Many of their hardships were the product of poverty and its associated injuries, coupled with the inability of the overburdened public hospital system to address their unique needs. The indifference of the broader community, along with the absence of social and religious support, also contributed to their misery. Remembering John Treeo, one wonders who among us is willing to cry for Mr. and Mrs. Wheeler and all the tens of thousands of "invisible" indigent persons who die each year in similar circumstances.

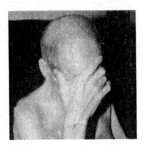

Chapter

7

A CONCLUSION: CONSCIOUS LISTENING, MINDFUL PRESENCE —A LESSON LEARNED

The inner-city dying poor have been the greatest teachers in my life. From listening to their stories, I have come to realize that presence is extremely important. In the Buddhist view of the world, there are two kinds of suffering—the kind that leads to more suffering and the kind that brings an end to suffering. Although dying is a form of suffering that ultimately ends with death, the weight of loss and grief hovering over dying persons and their loved ones is lifted by caring partnerships. When real care is present, it has a capacity to heal the spirit and render the dying whole. This care must encompass an integrated array of medical, nursing, psychosocial, community, and spiritual support. Its cornerstone is empathy, that is to say, an understanding of and appreciation for both the cultural milieu and the unique circumstances of each person's life. When patients and loved ones are isolated and abandoned by indifference, real care cannot be present, and thereby suffering is intensified. As Emily Dickinson wrote, "Pain prepares us for peace," but this peace can be fully realized only within connectedness to others. The centerpiece of connectedness with the dying poor is the ability to successfully imagine their world, putting oneself in their place. Thus, a major lesson demonstrated in these stories is the importance of conscious listening and mindful presence in bringing about an end to suffering. In fact, they would be, according to the principles of Buddhism, essential components in the liberation of the inner-city poor from their suffering at the end of life. They are also sources of enlightenment and learning for those of us in the broader community. Perhaps there is no more powerful articulation of the moral mandate to include the dying in our lives than the words of Dame Cicely Saunders:

> The dying need the community, its help, fellowship, care and attention, which will quiet their distress and fears and enable them to go peacefully. The community needs the dying to make it think of eternal issues and to make it listen and give to others.

First, I should summarize what I have learned about dying and about dying poor. Dying is one of the hardest challenges anyone faces in his or her life. Certainly, it is possible for the last stage of life to be meaningful and comfortable, but the incidence of this is all too rare. Poor communication between health-care providers and patients frequently leads to uncertainty and misunderstandings. Anger, fear, sadness, and guilt about losing one's own life or losing a loved one bring unparalleled stress and chaos to family life. The American tendency to ignore suffering and death leads to profound isolation for both dying persons and loved ones.

Although dying is incredibly difficult for every human being, the challenges faced by the poor are even greater. These individuals, who are among the most vulnerable, disempowered, and neglected in our society, experience unique chaos in many facets of their lives. They have trouble getting to their appointments, often because they do not own a car or have access to reliable transportation. They often do not understand their diseases and prognoses but are nevertheless called upon to make crucial decisions about their care. They face the physical debility common to all dying persons but do so in less comfortable surroundings: in three-story walk-up apartments, in homes with one bathroom on the second floor, in small and dark homes in bad neighborhoods, in condemned housing, in county-run nursing homes, and even under bridges. In addition, they face financial difficulties both related to and unrelated to their medical care. They also often experience dying in the context of chaotic family lives. All this chaos does not occur only in the hospital during the last days or weeks of life. In fact, a great deal of the stress occurs much earlier and extends well beyond the walls of the hospital into the home and community. Beyond these common features of dying and dying poor, it is clear from the narratives of dying individuals how each person's life story remains utterly unique and affects the experience of dying in ways impossible to predict.

Annie Dickens experienced God's power in ways that cannot be denied. God gave her the perseverance to endure bodily destruction and face death steadily. She lived her dying as an expression of her faith and as an opportunity to teach others about it. She suffered pain, could not eat, could not walk, and could not even get out of bed. Breathing was a struggle, as was finding the strength and breath to talk. Still, in the most dignified and grateful way, she presided over her dying with remarkable serenity. In this regard, Annie serves as a teacher offering lessons in life and demonstrating how faith provides hope and courage. Her spirit, never dampened despite her body being ravaged by disease, was sustained throughout dying by her unwavering belief in God's presence.

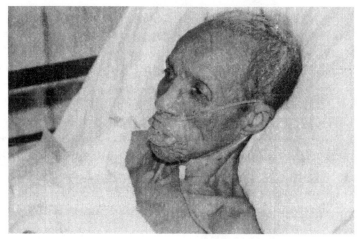

Annie Dickens: a profile in courage.

Mr. Wheeler filtered the experience of dying through anger and mistrust. Never escaping the economic pinch of being poor, he resented the lack of health-care options available to him. Unable to find solace in faith or social support, he became ironically dependent on the "curative powers" of doctors and a system he deeply resented. His feelings of disempowerment seemed to spin out of control in synchronization with the spread of his disease and the worsening of symptoms. As he awoke each day struggling for serenity and meaning, it was anger and bitterness that he experienced. These feelings of discontent, unique to him, were worn like a badge of honor. I often thought of how they provided him with a sense of individuality and empowerment. In a sense, to know Mr. Wheeler was to come to understand and accept that anger and distrust gave him a paradoxical fortitude and ability to endure his suffering. Thus, while his spirit was severely depressed throughout his illness, he was able to find ways of embracing life, even if

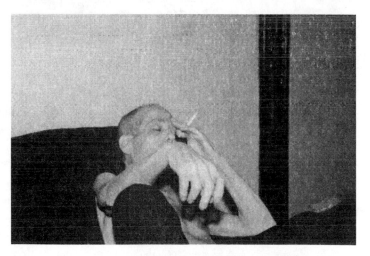

Mr. Wheeler: a survivor.

it was something as simple as eating spicy chicken wings. Although he knew they would make him sick, it was a means of maintaining control and independence in the face of loss.

The visage, physical strength, and mental toughness of "Big Sam" were apparent throughout the end-of-life experience of Joe Noble. One could almost feel how Joe's formidable strength and unassailable optimism had their roots in the harsh life experiences of his father in Russia, Canada, and the United States. Joe was angry, not at the fact that he was dying, but at the injuries imposed on his family by poverty. A deeply spiritual rather than religious man, he found comfort in the beauty of nature and the love of his family. These were the cornerstones of his life that, along with his immense resilience, enabled him to suffer the burden of serious long-term illness, economic deprivation, and prolonged dying with an air of nobility.

Dying in the county nursing home in an urban area, J. W. Green found comfort and meaning in lessons he learned in the rural South. An easy target of criticism for irresponsible behavior throughout his life, he was also a man exuberant in faith and was surprisingly sagacious about life. He understood the painful stigma of being poor in a culture of affluence and, unfortunately, suffered indignities in care because of his social and economic status. Nonetheless, he was able to transcend to a significant degree both the legacy of his reckless behavior on the city streets and the mistreatment in the nursing home. Dying peacefully, even heroically, all the while abandoning his sins and sufferings to God's love, his spirit and soul remained unbroken until the moment of death.

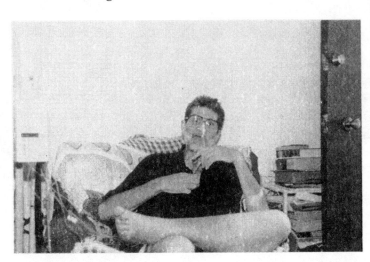

Joe Noble: teacher.

Virble and Ken suffered greatly and endured hardship after hardship, their tribulations steadily worsened by the grip of poverty. Living lives that seemed to have mattered so little to so many pursuing their own materialistic dreams, the Whites' experience in dying is a grievous reminder of the wretched epitaph of John Treeo. Perhaps, in judging Ken and Virble from afar, it is easy to dismiss them as losers in the competitive footrace of capitalism and the accumulation of material wealth. To get to know these individuals, however, was to witness them from a different vantage point, one that unveils the deepest and most cherished qualities of an enlightened, democratic society, namely, faithfulness, loyalty, hard work, perseverance, commitment, and love. Indeed, Ken and Virble offer a chilling test of the materialistic, self-centered values that drive so much of American life. In undeniable fashion, this loving

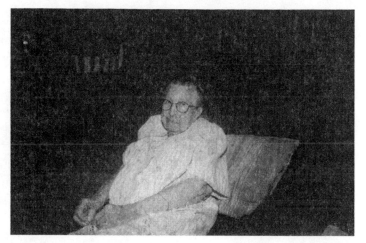

The Whites: loyalty and commitment through poverty.

couple, married for almost forty-four years, demonstrate to all of us where life's greatest joys and achievements may be found—and how they are not found within the materialistic dreams that drive so many. Their narrative also demonstrates the great injustice of the contemptible care they received as indigent patients in the nursing home, as well as the indignity wrought by not being able to pay for their funerals. Nonetheless, despite the harm they experienced because of their poverty, their spirit remained resolute and their love for each other indomitable.

Mrs. Angel's experience of dying was shaped by a particular pattern that she repeated again and again. She was a loving and gentle person and strove to be a good Christian woman and do what was expected of her. Her world, however, was often cruel. Her first husband physically abused her. He also psychologically abused their children. Her physicians and

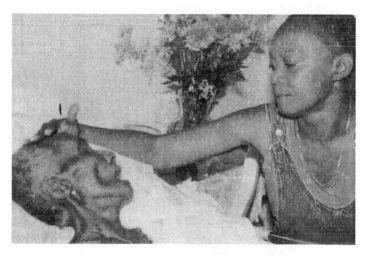

Mrs. Angel: beloved mother.

pastor during these years did not try to extricate her from this situation. Rather, they treated her symptoms and even implicitly placed blame on her. They gave her medicines so that she could get out of bed and tried to give her advice about how not to anger her husband. She regretted her weakness and the effects it had on her children. However, when she fought back against a cruel world—abusive husband, uncaring physician, cancer—she was wracked by guilt. Of what importance was her life that she should stand up for herself and demand others to care for her? It did not seem Christian. She thus tacked back and forth between feeling ashamed of her weakness and then of her strength. Nevertheless, she knew how to love others and took great pride in her children. Her daily prayers and arguments with God allowed her to persevere through her suffering, although she never understood if she brought it on herself or if it was just chance that brought so much suffering into her life. Nonetheless, her death was ultimately beautiful; a gift bestowed by her beloved daughters, who orchestrated a splendiferous symphony of caretaking during the final weeks of her life. In this ministry of love and partnership, the Angel family ultimately demonstrated their strength, spirit, heart, soul, and sisterly fellowship.

Throughout the lives of all the individuals featured in this book, two things remained constant: poverty and resilience. In many ways, as discussed earlier, resilience and strength are tethered to the experience of living poor. Thus, whether it be in the form of Mr. Wheeler's "self-expressive anger," Virble's devotion to Ken, Annie's profound faith, Joe's remarkable courage, or Mrs. Angel's dedication to her family, the spirit of many inner-city dying poor remains unbroken and breathes vitality into the soul and heart of their lives. In this way, the portrait that emerges in *Dancing with Broken Bones* is ultimately one of an unremitting strength and ruggedness that is reflective of the most virtuous ideals of the American character. It is truly a profile in courage from which there is much to learn, that is, if we can summon the fortitude to consciously listen to their stories and be mindfully present in their lives and throughout their deaths.

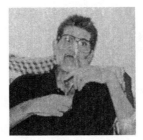

EPILOGUE:
AN URBAN THOREAU

A s the great twentieth-century philosopher Yogi Berra once said, "It's not over until it's over." Yogi's wisdom applies to many situations, whether it be a ball game, life itself, or the story of a person's life. It would thus be remiss if I did not complete the narrative of Cowboy. As noted earlier, there was much in his life that was grim: poverty, racism, mental illness, and estrangement from family. As I will show, there was much about the end of his life that was wonderful: support, good medical care, gratitude, and reconciliation.

Winter was rapidly approaching at the point I interrupted the story. Despite the fact that Cowboy had remained brazen in his attitude, his body was betraying him. Living in the cave was beginning to become unmanageable and even dangerous. For example, one night he suffered chest pains and was short of breath. Trying to get out of bed, he stumbled to the ground. In the dark on hands and knees, he crawled through the entrance of the cave, up the hill, and across the street to a public phone. He called 911 and collapsed onto the sidewalk. The emergency medical technicians arrived promptly, and within ten minutes or so Cowboy was at the emergency room of County, having suffered a heart attack. Although tests revealed that he had not suffered major damage to his heart, everyone was concerned about him going back home to live under the bridge, alone, in the dark, and with the weather turning cold. Therefore, Linda, still deeply committed to his care, was trying to find a place for him to live after he was discharged. With the assistance of a street minister, the same one who paid for the hotel room in which John Evans ("the grand old man of the ER") lived, she was able to arrange for a room at a

YMCA for two weeks. Grateful for her effort, Cowboy went there to stay after being discharged. It was situated about a mile from the cave, and he would go there each day to check on Cowgirl and enjoy the familiarity of his home.

The room, being close to the campus, enabled Linda to pick him up and drive him to his medical appointments. Most of the time he would be waiting for her arrival, but there were a few occasions when he did not show up. Frankly, Cowboy was always happiest when immersed in street life. Thus, if the spirit moved him or if a "better offer" presented itself, he would go off to gamble, see friends, or return to the cave. Linda would wait for him, agitated and often thinking, "What are we going to do with this guy?" At first when this would happen, she felt not only frustrated but also disrespected. As she was discovering, her relationship with Cowboy was complicated and challenged her both professionally and personally. The palliative care medical director answered her question directly: "We will love him until he dies." Despite his occasional irresponsibility, that was exactly what she committed to do. However, loving Cowboy was no small challenge. Made difficult not only by his long-term inability to receive or give love but by his unstable mental state as well, caring for this man required special patience. It was energy and time consuming, and often put her to the test.

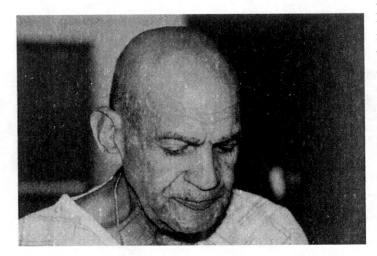

A quiet reflection about living and dying.

"We would constantly do this dance together where he would push me away and then seek me out," she said. Cowboy could not allow her to get too close. His capacity for intimacy and closeness had been kidnapped long ago in Mississippi.

The first week at the Y went smoothly. Cowboy continued to visit the cave regularly by bus or bicycle. On Thursday afternoons I would pick him up with a group of medical students, and we would go there together for a "home visit." These visits were always appreciated. He praised the students for their dedication and commitment to becoming physicians. He told jokes, and invariably, when he described how he sometimes shined shoes for a living, he would look down at someone's feet and say, "It looks like those could use a little work." Still persuasive and forceful in his personality, a befuddled intern or medical student would have little choice but to remove a shoe. Cowboy would shine it with "spit and polish," while continuing to share the story of his life. He took great pride in this work, and to everyone's surprise, the shoeshine would be really good. Despite the weakening of this body, he was still full of piss and vinegar, especially when presenting his views on racial matters.

His rage and anger at his family, including his children, seemed little affected by the toll the disease was taking on his body. During my relationship with him, I had come to learn that Cowboy, in many ways, needed to be angry. Having been so deeply injured as a child, anger was one way of responding to the cruelty he endured. For the students not used to such outbursts, these visits were eye opening. For most of their training they saw patients in a very narrow, clinical way and seldom in their own environments, and few were so expressive about profoundly personal matters. John, a first year intern, perhaps put it best when he said, "Thank you for the privilege of getting to meet and know this man." Just as importantly, the benefits of these visits were mutual. They were

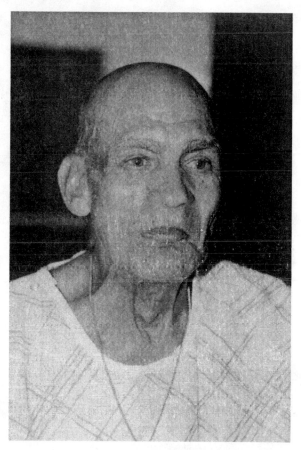

Playful talk about the loves of his life: Cowgirl and Linda.

valuable for Cowboy in letting him know he mattered. They showed him that there were people who cared enough to visit and listen to his life story.

During this time Cowgirl remained faithfully at the cave awaiting his return each day. I checked on her regularly to ensure that she had enough food and water. Ironically, despite prolonged periods of being empty, the cave and its contents remained undisturbed. How unlikely, I thought, that its contents had not been stolen or vandalized.

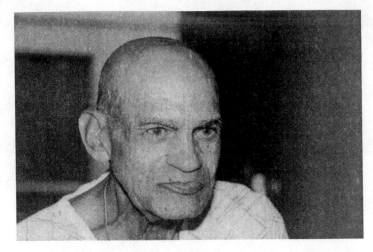

The familiar look of mischief returns as he feels better.

Unfortunately, despite the good things that were happening, Cowboy's living situation was becoming problematic. He was often unable and unwilling to follow the house rules at the Y. The problem peaked one day when he decided that he did not like the stained white walls of his room, so he went out, got some paint, and began redecorating. A room inspection revealed that the walls and radiator had been spray-painted bright red. Cowboy was to be evicted. He seemed not to care. He would just go back to the cave, but Linda worried that if he returned there he would be in real trouble. He was continuing to fail physically, and the temperature was dropping into the single digits at night. By pleading with the manager, she was able to convince him to let Cowboy stay one more night. In the meantime she tried to find somewhere else for him to stay. Essentially unperturbed by the situation, Cowboy told her not to worry and that he would be fine. Having come to love him as she did, she did worry. Once again she went to work on finding a place for him, but he kept insisting that, "You can't worry about these things more than I do."

Sometimes good news emerges from misfortune. The next day before the hour of eviction, Cowboy's breathing dif-

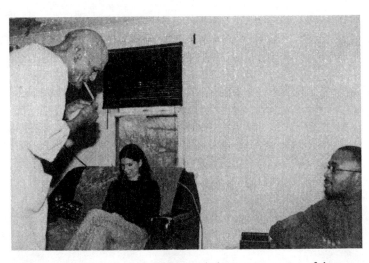

In his new digs Cowboy continues to teach the next generation of doctors.

ficulties worsened. He was rushed to the emergency room. His pain had intensified, his bowels were failing, and he was in acute respiratory distress. The bad news was that he needed to be admitted to the hospital. That, however, was also the good news, because Linda, despite diligent efforts, had not been able to locate a place for him to stay. His admission provided her with more time. The other part of the good news was that the medical interns who had gotten to know him through home visits were now back working on the wards at County. Having grown intrigued by and fond of this man, they were all exceptionally dedicated to his care. Thus, under the direction of Dr. G. and Jodi, Cowboy received exemplary medical care. A private room had been arranged. He was settling down, becoming more comfortable, and regaining some strength. It was at this point that I sensed a major transformation in both his attitude and spirit. His seemingly intractable veneer of anger was starting to soften. For the first time, he seemed to be capable of allowing others to take care of him without resisting. Slowly, he was becoming less suspicious and more trusting as his heart was opening just a bit.

I jokingly refer to Linda as the World Wrestling Federation social worker. Seemingly, there is never a problem, no matter how unusual or complicated, that she cannot grasp hold of and "body slam" with resolution for patients and families. While Cowboy was in the hospital, she had been hard at work to find a new place for him to live. It paid off. She was able to locate a small apartment that rented for $250 a month. It was a run-down, roach-infested walk-up in the heart of an inner-city neighborhood known for drugs, gangs, and violence. Even so, it was warm, and he would be safe. Grateful and glad to be there, Cowboy felt comfortably at home in his new place. He immediately went to work on attacking the roach problem by devising traps made of bleach and water. His spirit was strong. Cowgirl was with him, having been brought from the cave on the day he was discharged. Thursday afternoon visits with medical students continued, and although his body was being weakened by disease, he remained independent and joyful.

Unfortunately, this new living situation did not last long. Cowboy and Linda had met with the landlady's son to make arrangements for the apartment. He paid, with Linda as a witness, $250 for a security deposit and another $250 for the first month's rent. This person, who was a drug abuser and dealer, absconded with the money. (Subsequently, he disappeared entirely and was thought to have been murdered. The detectives assigned to the case recently gave this news to his mother.) Having received neither rent money nor security deposit, the landlady decided to evict Cowboy. Linda tried to intervene. She assured her that Cowboy had paid the money in full to her son, but the landlady would not be persuaded. Pursuing the matter, Linda pleaded with her to let him stay. However, she remained steadfast in her decision, stating that it was not only about the money, but that, "He's going to die, and I don't want him lying dead on the floor above me." Once again, Cowboy was without a place to stay.

Linda was becoming frustrated at how time consuming her relationship with Cowboy had become. Expressing this frustration to Dr. G., she vented, "I just don't know what to do for him anymore." Dr. G. repeated what was now becoming a driving mantra of the team's involvement with Cowboy: "We are going to love him until he dies."

Loving him remained difficult. In fact, Linda had already been criticized by medical students for allowing Cowboy to manipulate and exploit her. At this point she had already invested more than 100 hours in his care. Nonetheless, having grown to love this man as a unique person, she was not about to abandon him, regardless of the demands placed on her. So once again, driven by compassion and the duty to serve, she went to work on finding Cowboy suitable housing. She was able to secure placement in the transitional residence for homeless men discharged from the hospital. Cowboy would be allowed to stay for thirty days, providing he obeyed the house rules. He got off to a reasonably good start, but problems emerged. It is not difficult to understand that obeying rules was not Cowboy's forte, nor would it ever be. His transgressions were not egregious enough to get him evicted this time. Rather, he pushed the envelope sufficiently to become "beloved but difficult," in the words of the house director. He would play his music too loud on occasion, would be late for curfew, and would not always follow the protocol for kitchen behavior. Clearly, he was violating house rules, but the staff felt that they would be able to work productively with him and be successful in nudging him toward greater compliance. However, while Cowboy seemed to be successfully walking the tightrope of acceptable behavior, misfortune once again struck. The spread of his disease was beginning to compromise his bowels. Almost overnight Cowboy became incontinent. Thus, the same rule that forced Ernest to move from the Gilead House to Deerfield Village led to his eviction.

After being evicted, Cowboy disappeared and was nowhere to be found. Later we discovered that he had spent some time with a lady friend, spent a night in the back of a car, and stayed with friends at a local underground gambling establishment known as the pea shake house. During his shuffle, Cowgirl disappeared.

We saw him for the first time two weeks later. Cowboy was brought to the emergency room; his pain was elevated, his bowels were not functioning, and he was in respiratory distress. Again he was admitted to the hospital, making this the tenth hospitalization in three months. The pain in his back was intense and made it difficult for him to lie in bed. He spent much of his time sitting, heavily sedated by morphine. He drifted off to sleep regularly and often seemed in danger of falling out of the chair. He knew he was getting sicker and that the end of his life was nearing. He respectfully spoke about God and welcomed the spiritual ministry of the palliative care team chaplain. Medical residents and students continued to look in on him. He remained grateful for their visits. His anger was continuing to dissipate and he was experiencing an unfamiliar but well-deserved sense of peace and equanimity.

As the days passed his body continued to be ravaged by disease. Nonetheless, because his medical care remained exemplary, the physical agony was minimized. Additionally, perhaps for the only time in his life, he was being nourished by love.

How strange, I thought, that in dying Cowboy was finally finding a sense of comfort that had eluded him throughout life. His major regret at this point was that he feared that Cowgirl was dead. "I think I've lost Cowgirl," he pined with tears welling in his eyes. He went on to remark, "That's okay, because we will see each other again one day." He was referring to the two of them meeting in heaven.

On the morning of December 26, 2001, I called Cowboy in his hospital room. I began the conversation by saying, "Cowboy, there is someone I want to bring by to see you." "Who is it?" he asked. "Fannie," I said. "Aunt Fannie?" he queried. As it turned out, Linda, during one of her many efforts on his behalf, had stumbled across an aunt who raised Marvin for three years in Mississippi. As we were about to learn, before sending him away permanently when he was 13, Marvin's mother moved from the plantation for three years and left her son behind with her sister. Aunt Fannie raised him from years five through eight. Al-

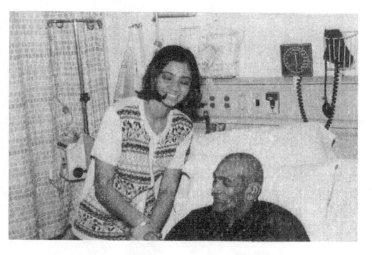

A most unusual partnership: bridging the divide between inner-city poor and student–physicians.

though they were mostly estranged throughout his adult life, Fannie had made her way to Indianapolis. Coincidentally, she was living less than a mile from the cave.

His response seemed like an epiphany. "Okay. I trust you," he answered. I was particularly stunned when he went on to add, "Don't worry, I'll behave myself." Finally, Cowboy's soul was beginning to find comfort. In the process of dying, he was opening to reconciliation, forgiveness, and fellowship. Vitriol and anger were being left behind almost as if he knew they would be intolerable baggage in the place that lay ahead for him.

On December 26, Linda and I brought Fannie, now eighty years old, to see her nephew. There was no antagonism or tension in sight as they reminisced about their lives and relationship. Things were off to a good start, and after five minutes I seized the opportunity to push the matter further, saying, "Cowboy, with your permission, I'd like to see if we can arrange something else." "What's that?" he replied. "I think it's time to see your children." It was as if he had been anticipating what I had in mind. Showing neither surprise nor anger, he simply said, "I'd like to see them." The communication between us had been clear. Linda now had permission to locate the children, and a reunion, perhaps even reconciliation, might take place. Cowboy immediately returned his attention to the conversation that Linda and Fannie were having, and, of course, being the uncontrollable flirt he was, the discussion inevitably drifted toward "the way" he had with the ladies. "Even as a young boy, he was a 'real charmer,'" Fannie confided. The visit lasted forty-five minutes and was richly satisfying for both nephew and aunt. As we drove her home after the visit, Fannie said, "Thank you. It was good to see my nephew."

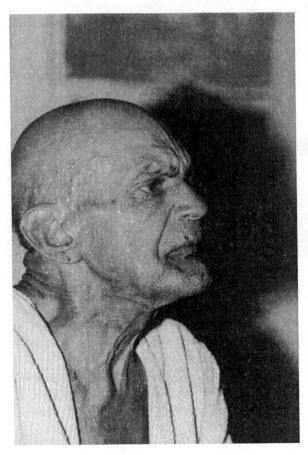

Lamenting the loss of Cowgirl.

The last time Michael Smith had seen his father was twenty years before. They inadvertently bumped into each other outside a variety store in an inner-city neighborhood. Upon recognizing his son, Cowboy instinctually recoiled and snarled, "I never gave a fuck about you!" His venom in spewing these words was consistent with the psychoemotional damage he suffered as a child. However, even though Cowboy had bolted from his son's life years ago, Michael nevertheless loved his father and felt the sting of those words deeply. For profoundly complex reasons, Cowboy could relate to his children only as he was raised: hurtfully and spitefully.

Even though I had previously not known the depth of the estrangement between father and son, I understood fully that the rift was bad. For this reason it was indeed shocking that on December 28, hours after having been contacted by Linda, Michael arrived at his father's bedside. A lot had happened in Michael's life. After having graduated from Ohio State University and completing his graduate work at Harvard, he was drawn back to the city streets. Already damaged emotionally and mentally, "It was the only place I knew to go," he confessed. His life for the past thirty years had not been productive from the point of view of prevailing cultural values. He worked infrequently and lived in poverty. A spiritual quest to the city of Touba in Senegal had led him to convert to Islam. No longer Michael, he was now Sheik Ibrahim.

Frankly, the reunion was largely uneventful. There was too much to be said that could not be said. Cowboy was too sick and the issues too deep. Their interaction went smoothly, if superficially, with Ibrahim internalizing his emotions. While there he happened to look into the closet in the hospital room and was horrified by the condition of his father's clothes. They were sooty, dingy, and tattered. Perhaps the only proud memory he had was of the way his father dressed and presented himself. You will remember Cowboy had described this as "cash and flash—flash and cash." In fact, when Marvin was living in Chicago he was named Best-Dressed Black Man by a local black organization on two separate occasions. It was on seeing and smelling his father's clothes that Ibrahim came to learn that he had lived for the past three years under a bridge. He was upset by how poverty and mental illness had shattered the one memory of his father he could recall without regret. At that moment in the hospital room, Ibrahim was gripped by fear and revulsion. He quickly told his father he needed to leave but would be back to see him soon.

Perhaps there is no more awful death than to die with regret, feeling that one's life has been wasted. Perhaps there can be no greater sentence imposed on one's future than to witness the death of a loved one when there is grave and irreconcilable emotional disrepair.

In this regard, for Cowboy, death seemed not so horrible because of his faith in God and because he felt satisfied with his life. For better or for worse, despite unimaginable youthful injuries, he had lived life on his own terms. Although he suffered greatly and passed his pain on to his children, he was able to maintain his own style and individuality throughout his life. He had lived with passion, enjoying women, music, work, and fashion. He often impressed others with his zest for life. "I will remember Marvin as a man of charm, wit, intelligence, and one who appreciated fashion and complimented style," remarked Barbara, the palliative care team chaplain. Death seemed not so horrible to Cowboy because he had found ways to live without regret and had embraced the possibilities of the life he had been granted.

Maybe most impressive is the fact that at age sixty-five he had received his GED. Throughout his life he had been resentful of being deprived of an education. As you will recall, he was told he was "too stupid to learn." Cowboy took pride in his vocabulary and his ability to enunciate difficult words and displayed an enthusiasm for learning. Thus, as he spoke about this accomplishment, I sensed that it was almost as if to snub his nose at his family that he had gotten his high school equivalency diploma. He took delight in the achievement, certainly, but also enjoyed "sticking it in their faces." Additionally, Cowboy was always well respected by his peers, who saw him as honest, intelligent, and witty. On the streets he was known as "the mayor," a title bestowed precisely because of these qualities. In short, as his anger and excitability were waning in the nurturing arms of a caring group of professionals, Cowboy was at a place where he could review his life with minimum regret and begin to feel a sense of peace.

The challenge before Ibrahim, however, was quite different. There was nothing peaceful about being reunited with his dying father. It rekindled painful thoughts about neglect and abuse. Not only had Cowboy affected his life in hurtful ways, but his death would eliminate any possibility of reconciliation. There may be no greater expression of the pain Ibrahim felt throughout his life than the words of a poem he wrote in 1982, pain brought about by being poor in a culture of affluence and black in a racist society, the injuries of which were exacerbated through abandonment and rejection by his father.

> What about the rape of our body,
> What about the rape of our mind,
> What about the rape of our time,
> What about the rape of our dream,
> What about the rape of our love.

In 1998, while estranged from Cowboy, Ibrahim had self-published a collection of poetry entitled *Invocation for the Mentally Insane, Excerpt Poems for the Lost and Found*. Despite the fact he had not seen his father for seventeen years, he wrote the following words of special thanks in the acknowledgment section: "to My Father, (A Surviving King)." Throughout the years of exile from his father, Ibrahim yearned for connection. His heart remained conflicted between rage and anger toward him and the need to love and forgive. Tension between those emotions would never be more pressing than at this particular point in his life.

Ibrahim remained true to his word and returned to see his father the following day. He brought with him a newly purchased shirt and pair of shoes. "I just cannot bear the thought of my father wearing those clothes," he remarked. Although he seemed to understand that Cowboy would never be well enough to wear his new outfit, "at least he would have something decent to be buried in," Ibrahim stated. At this point, he was unaware that months before Cowboy had decided against a funeral for several reasons, one of which was the belief that "No one would come," and that "If people are interested in seeing me, let them do it while I'm alive."

During this period, Dwight, Cowboy's other son, also came to visit. Having worked for a local affiliate of CBS, he was now a pastor in Dayton, Ohio. Dwight had been estranged from Cowboy off and on for most of his life. They had had a major falling out many years ago and had not seen each other since. When Dwight had sought to contact him just the previous year, their paths unfortunately never crossed. When first contacted by Linda, Dwight was in shock. He had come to think his father was probably dead. Hearing that he was still alive was startling and opened a floodgate of conflicting emotions, anger, and confusion. Nonetheless, true to his ministry as a Christian pastor and driven by a personal need to find reconciliation, he arrived at Cowboy's bedside on December 28. He came alone and in secret. The situation was so bad that he could not even tell his mother what he was up to, as this ex-wife and Cowboy were bitterly estranged. As he walked into the room on the sixth floor and saw his now dying father for the first time in years, the experience was overwhelming: wounds were reopened, and a painful intensity ensued. However, their conversation was amicable. The past was not brought up, and Cowboy was pleased to see his son. Dwight stayed for about an hour and then left to travel back to Ohio. He drove in deep reflection about the anticipated loss of his presumed-dead father and their embittered relationship.

Cowboy was in a different state of mind. Having gotten to a peaceful place in his life, seeing his sons did not have a significant emotional impact on him. He simply enjoyed their visits. On the other hand, for Ibrahim and Dwight, the emotional consequence was huge. Feelings that had been deeply buried were stirred. As a result, they were psychoemotionally shaken by their encounters. In response, they individually retreated to their private lives, Dwight to his ministry in Dayton and Ibrahim to the solitude of the reclusive spiritual journey he had been on for the past two years. They would not see their father again for seventeen days. Unfortunately, Linda was unable to locate Cowboy's daughter, who was reportedly living in Chicago at this point, so a reunion between Shirlene and her father did not take place.

In the meantime, insurance regulations required that Cowboy be discharged from the hospital. The residents had already delayed discharging him because they knew he had nowhere to go. Unable to justify hospitalization any longer, Cowboy was transferred to the nursing home. Deerfield Village would become his final residence before death. He knew he was dying. Be that as it may, thanks to good control of pain and other symptoms, he was still able to enjoy life. He paid off all his debts, most of which were from money borrowed from friends or gambling associates. He reveled in the love displayed by the palliative care team. He quickly became a favorite of the health service professionals who worked on his floor at Deerfield. He was not bothered by the fact that his sons had not returned to visit nor bothered to call. Instead, he focused on positive things: his love of women (especially Linda), his favorite music, and his unwavering belief in God. In a strange way, this was a good time for both Cowboy and those who cared for him.

Over the next three weeks, things remained pretty much the same. Cowboy enjoyed being the center of attention at Deerfield. Although they had not known him long, many of the staff came to care deeply about this "interesting" and "cool" man. None of his children were involved. We still had not been able to track down his daughter, and his sons had not returned. Cowboy gave this no thought whatsoever. Friends from the neighborhood would visit, including Dr. Ralph of the federally funded Homeless Initiative Program. "I'd visit and we'd talk about music. Cowboy loved jazz," Ralph said.

Occasionally, if he were feeling up to it, someone would take him out for a while, back to the streets where he felt most at home: to look for Cowgirl, to say hello to friends, perhaps to stop at Burger King for a cup of coffee. During these weeks, there were two constants in his life: the progression of his disease and the abiding love of those at County whose lives he touched. Cowboy, often alone in life, was now befriended in dying.

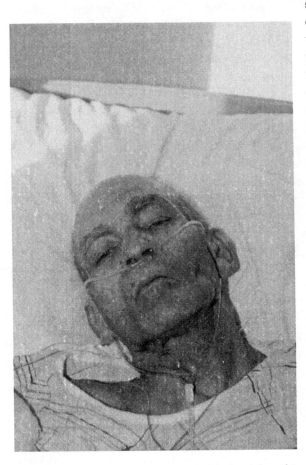

Peace, love, and gratitude were deeply felt throughout his final days in the nursing home.

On Thursday, January 10, Linda and I were riding back to campus after having participated in a community presentation about caring for the dying poor at County. After our talk, at which we told a bit of the story of Cowboy, the first question asked was, "What happened to the dog?" We explained that she had been missing then for six weeks and was feared dead. Multiple attempts to find her at the pound and in the neighborhoods had been unsuccessful. We mentioned that Cowboy grieved and cried over her loss but felt confident that they would "see each other again someday." Later, as Linda and I continued talking about the enthusiastic response of the audience, an idea occurred.

"We don't have to rush back. Let's take one more drive though the neighborhood," I said, so we drove to the cave and then up Martin Luther King, Jr., Street to the apartment where Cowboy had briefly lived before being evicted. We were looking for Cowgirl as we circled the streets. Not surprisingly, she could not be found, but maybe Yogi knew what he was talking about after all. As we searched, one final thought occurred. "Let's check with the landlady about the dog," I suggested. Linda, a bit concerned, asked, "Do you think she'll talk to us?"

"All she can say is no."

"Let's do it," she decided.

We rang the bell and were graciously received by Mrs. M. She talked painfully about how her son was missing and presumed dead. She elaborated on her faith and reliance on God throughout this difficult time. We hesitated to inquire about Cowgirl, as her disappearance paled in comparison to this mother's grief. Nonetheless, we asked and she responded, "Oh yes, I see her everyday at 5:30."

"At night?" we queried.

"No, I feed her every morning at 5:30, and then she goes off."

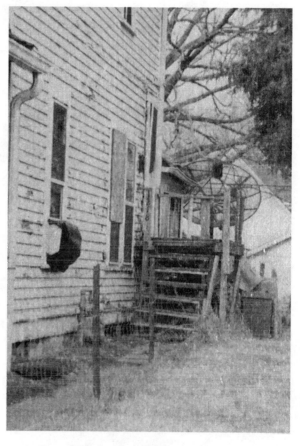

Cowgirl would wait patiently for Cowboy's return until she was abused and injured.

Unbelievable, we thought, Cowgirl is alive! As it turned out, day after day she sat outside the door waiting for Cowboy to return after his eviction. Mrs. M. began feeding her at that point. When the apartment was rented shortly thereafter, the new tenant did not like the dog hanging around, and he kicked her, injuring a hip. As a result Cowgirl would come to the house to be fed early in the morning but would wander off soon thereafter to avoid further abuse. Stunned by the news that she was still alive, we knew we had one more challenge in front of us. We needed to find and retrieve Cowgirl.

On Sunday, January 13, we went back to the neighborhood and began our search. As if it were supposed to happen, we found Cowgirl almost immediately. She appeared bigger, having grown, and her hair was thickened by the winter weather. She was also frightened and hurt. We were able to corral her in a backyard. She was trepidacious but not aggressive. Cowboy had once told me, "She doesn't like most people, but now that she knows you, she'll never hurt you. Nope, she won't." Talking gently to her, I tried to approach slowly. It took one hour and forty-five minutes before I was able to get a leash around her. Getting her into a car was just as difficult, but we persisted and finally succeeded.

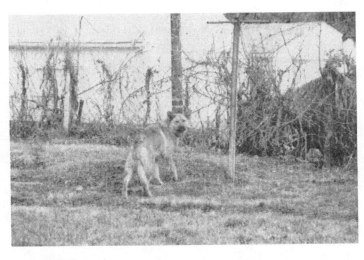
Cowgirl frightened.

Joining us were Peggy, a respiratory therapist at Deerfield Village, and her husband, Tom. When Peggy, who is an animal rescuer, learned that Cowgirl was alive she offered to take her in and find her a foster home. During the effort to get Cowgirl into Peggy's truck, a nurse at Deerfield paged Linda. Cowboy had taken a dramatic turn for the worse, and it seemed that death would not be far away. Linda went on to the nursing home to be with him. Peggy, Tom, and I continued our struggle with Cowgirl.

Once we got her inside the truck, we drove straight to the nursing home. Cowgirl was resistant but not aggressive as we dragged her into the building, onto the elevator, and down the fourth-floor hallway into Cowboy's room. As soon as she saw him, she sprang to life. She rushed to him, climbed onto the bed, and lay across his chest. Licking his face and hands, she aroused Cowboy. Weakly opening his eyes, he smiled and put his arm around her, saying, "Cowgirl's here!"

Over the next two hours, many of the staff roamed into the room. News of this event had even spread to other floors, and people wanted to have a look. The general sentiment was perhaps best expressed by a nurse who said, "Amazing. Just amazing." Dr. Ralph stopped in to say good-bye to his friend. Barbara came as well to offer spiritual support. I went to pick up Fannie, who sat quietly by his side throughout. Before leaving she bent over, kissed him, and said, "I love you, Marvin." Tears were streaming down her cheeks. There was a real gathering of community at Marvin's bedside, a tribute to

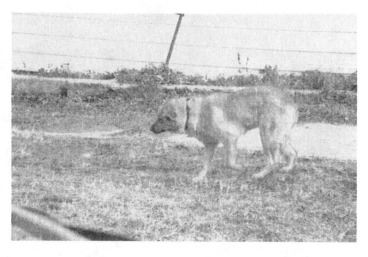

Showing her injury.

the capacity of this man to touch our lives. Around 5:00 on Sunday afternoon, Peggy left with Cowgirl, who eagerly went with her following the smell of Cowboy's slippers and pajamas. Linda and I kissed him and promised to return in the morning.

We arrived around 8:00 AM the next day. Dr. G. was already there, having brought a cup of coffee. Cowboy was able to take a few sips, and the nurse practitioner sighed, "It's all about pleasure at this point." Barbara came to pray. All of his physical needs, especially relief from respiratory distress and pain, were well attended to by the nursing staff. Death was imminent, but given the extent of his physical decline, he was remarkably peaceful. Around noon Linda and I needed to leave. I kissed him on the forehead, saying, "Thank you for being my friend, Cowboy." He managed a smile. It was now time for

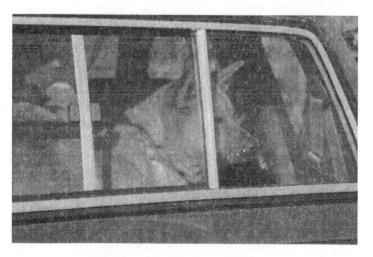

Now safe.

Linda to say goodbye to her dear friend. "Marvin, I have something for you," she said, arousing him. "It's what you always wanted." With grace and ease, she leaned over and kissed him on the lips. Their eyes met briefly, and he uttered what were to be his final words: "Thank you. I loved that."

We knew that Cowboy would soon be dead, and Linda went off to call Dwight and Ibrahim. She informed them that if they wanted to see their father before he died, they had best come immediately. They did, returning for the first time since the initial reunion. Cowboy was unconscious by then, and he never knew that they spent several hours with him that night.

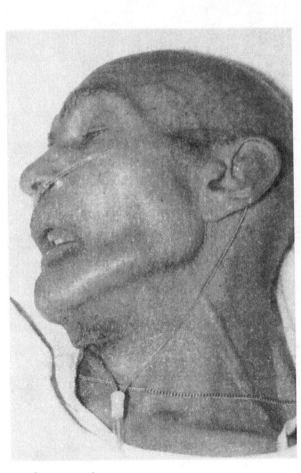

Cowboy worsening.

The next day I went to see Cowboy around 6:45 AM. There was a group of people milling around the nurses station, and as soon as I got off the elevator I knew something was up. Cowboy had died in his sleep at 1:55 AM on Tuesday, January 15, 2002. I called Linda to tell her the news. The nurses, other staff, and I lingered together for a while. They offered their remembrances, and I shared with them pictures of the reunion with Cowgirl that had taken place on Sunday. After ten minutes, they scurried off to their respective duties. I went down to his now-empty room with a reporter I had brought to meet him. Together we sat in the dark, and I reminisced about our relationship, offering suggestions as to why so many people were drawn to him. Despite great sadness, I felt joy in being a part of this uncommon experience, and I felt pride in how Cowboy had been so well served by the professionals at County.

I can only imagine that as he climbed the stairway to heaven, he was greeted by St. Peter, who applauded, saying, "Hey, Cowboy! Great death!" Perhaps St. Peter followed up with, "Now it's time to talk a bit about your life."

Linda had notified Ibrahim and Dwight of their father's death, and the four of us were scheduled to meet at 2:00 PM that afternoon. Their dominant feelings at this point were gratitude and confusion. They were thankful for the good care that Cowboy had received, especially finding comfort that so many different in-dividuals had taken an in-terest in their father. Their confusion was essentially overwhelming, however. Theirs was a unique and especially burdensome grief, and they felt the sting of a tidal wave of painful emo-tions that swept over them. They were suffering the loss of their father; a fa-ther they never really knew. Moreover, they were remembering in-stances of neglect and abusive treatment, and they were glaringly re-minded of how they suf-fered all those years. Their struggle was to grieve the death of a father who was never capable of loving them but whose love they so desperately needed.

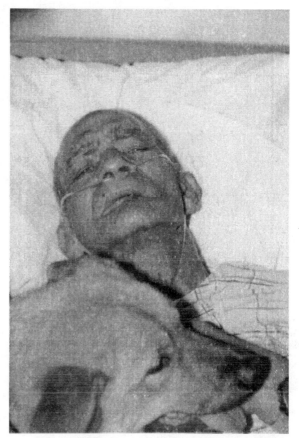

A reunion sooner than expected.

Dwight began. "My fa-ther grew up in the South?" I was stunned. I never imagined the separation between father and children had been so severe that they did not even know his birthplace. "Yes," I replied, "in Mississippi." I went on to describe his experi-ences as a boy and the recent circumstances of his life in the cave. All the while I was thinking to myself that Linda and I knew Cowboy far better than they did. How sad.

Both Ibrahim and Dwight were hungry for information and details. Any bit of knowledge that would help them make a connection with their father was appreciated. They hung on every word with anticipation that something might be revealed that would provide understanding and meaning. We showed pictures, which they passed back and forth as if they were sacred objects. Ibrahim seemed especially

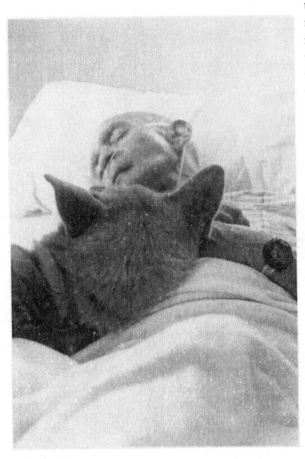

Solace and peace.

frightened. "I worry that I am going to wind up like this myself one day." A few tearful moments later it was as if a lightbulb had turned on. "You know, there's a man at Harvard who went off and lived in isolation. His name was Henry David Thoreau. What I see here in my father is Thoreau." "An urban Thoreau?" I inquired. "Exactly. Except that Henry David would leave Harvard and go to Walden Pond by choice. My father never had a choice. He never had the opportunity to attend Harvard as I did, and the circumstances of his life led him to live like this." Ibrahim was carving out a strategy for coping with the tragedy of Cowboy's life and death. In doing so he would filter his suffering through the image of his father as a creative and irrepressible rebel who lived his life as a form of protest.

Dwight, on the other hand, was struggling to comprehend the loss and pain as a Christian minister. He indicated that just the past Sunday he had given a sermon entitled "Dancing with Broken Bones." He turned directly to Ibrahim and spoke to him about how their father lived and danced with broken bones. Tears streamed down his cheeks. In this conversation he was trying to cope with his father's transgressions by forgiveness and understanding, an understanding based on coming to recognize for the first time that much of Marvin's irresponsibility as a father had been produced by the injuries he suffered as a boy. To this day, Dwight is still working on forgiveness.

After four emotionally draining hours, Ibrahim asked where Cowboy's body was and if he could see it. Linda made a phone call and alerted the morgue that we were coming. Dwight wanted to walk with us but waited outside while Linda, Ibrahim, and I went inside. Reverently, Ibrahim knelt beside his father's body. He began. "Father, I know you can hear me." He then proceeded to talk to and pray for him in both English and Arabic. All the while he was gently touching his father, as if to hold on to a connection that had never existed. After ten minutes, he kissed Cowboy on the forehead and gently zipped up the body bag. The three of us went outside to rejoin Dwight. Dwight and Ibrahim left the hospital to return to their respective homes.

Linda and I hugged goodbye, each of us going off to reflect on the impact Cowboy had made on our lives.

The first of two memorial services was held at noon on Wednesday. Staff from the Homeless Initiative Project and Deerfield Village gathered at the cave for a twenty-minute ceremony. There were several police officers

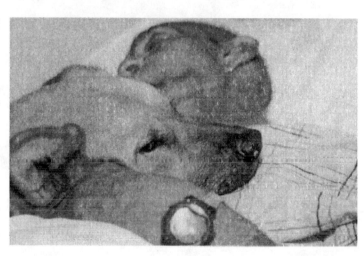

Best friends sleeping together for two hours while all the fourth-floor staff looked in on "the amazing sight."

in attendance, cops who were fond of Cowboy and protected him. Two of them had tears in their eyes as they told about their relationship. "He was a remarkable man," Officer Terri noted. "We always would keep an eye out for him." I finally understood why the cave would remain undisturbed when Cowboy was absent. The word on the street was not to mess with it, and the cops really did look after him. In fact, they visited almost every day, making the cave a "protected site." Thinking about how Cowboy had formed and creatively used these relationships to secure his survival brought a quiet smile to my face. All those years ago in Mississippi, he had learned how to survive by cultivating relationships with those who could help him. That very ability, which he developed as a boy, continued to serve him until the very end.

A local TV station had gotten wind of Cowboy's story and decided to cover the memorial service. In fact, as the news spread the media became quite interested in this uncommon life story. Five television spots, two of which were the lead story, and two newspaper columns appeared over the next five days. How ironic. Cowboy, so invisible in life as thousands of people drove over and past his home every day without regard for him, was becoming a celebrity of sorts in death. Too bad he wasn't there to see the outpouring of interest in the community. Frankly, he would have loved it.

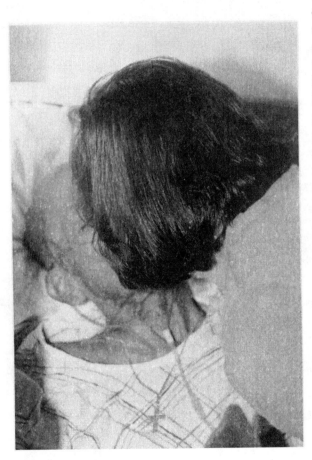

Linda says farewell to her dear friend.

The next day I took Terrence, the first year medical student who regularly saw Cowboy, on a bereavement visit to see Ibrahim. We picked Cowboy's son up at his home on the east side of the city. Because Ibrahim wanted to see where his father had lived, we headed downtown to the cave. A television reporter and camera crew were scheduled to meet us there at 3:00 PM.

Ibrahim entered the car in a somber mood. After exchanging hellos, he quickly began talking about Thoreau. Opening a portfolio filled with papers, he proceeded to read a passage from Thoreau's book *Civil Disobedience*. His voice trembled with anger as he continued reading. "This is my father. This is my father," he fumed, referring to the dehumanizing impact of the state and political economy to which he believed his father had fallen victim. Ibrahim's mind was whirling in the heavens and stars with ideas that legitimized his father's suffering and lifestyle. In this journey he was struggling to explain his father's life and searching for meaning to his own emotional pain. "My father's soul is not at peace," he lamented. "We are going to have to set it free." Terrence and I listened carefully, assuring him that Cowboy had been wonderfully cared for in the preceding months. In addition, we assured him that we had both noticed that a transformation had occurred. For the first time in his life, Cowboy had been able to acknowledge love. I went on to add that I believed that Cowboy's soul was at peace because of the warming fires of fellowship that saw him into his death. Ibrahim, still agitated, was not convinced.

We arrived at the cave, and the news crew was waiting. I told Ibrahim about the first time I had met Cowboy and how he had brought gifts out to Linda and me on the hill. I joked about how he was cleanly shaven and sporting a nice-smelling cologne, which I came to realize later was for Linda's benefit, not mine. Slowly, we went down the hill and entered through the plastic tarp. Ibrahim seemed mesmerized by the sight. Slowly, he walked from place to place, gently touching items at random. He was overwhelmed by what he saw, and the feelings engendered were shaking him visibly. Still struggling to make sense of his father's life, he announced to the reporter that on January 22, which would have been Cowboy's seventy-fourth birthday, he would begin a hunger fast to bring attention to the predicament of the homeless in Indianapolis. It would be in four parts: ten days of fruit, then ten days of juice, ten days of water, and the last ten days he would consume nothing but air. He invited the reporter to cover the fast. Shana said she would think about it.

The second memorial service was held on Saturday. About sixty people were in attendance, including Cowboy's daughter and Ibrahim's mother. The palliative care team was there, as were some students and friends of Cowboy from the community. Some who had never even met him came. They had been moved to attend by the stories in the media. Linda and I gave eulogies, and Dr. G. read from the scripture. As I spoke about Cowboy, I lit a black candle in front of the memorial board to symbolize the dark side of his life: poverty, racism, emotional damage, alienation, and mental illness. I concluded by asking Linda to join me and played the song "Cowboy, Take Me Away." We stood, arms around each other, listening to the words and saying good-bye to a dear friend.

Dwight spoke next and focused on the value of forgiveness. Then Ibrahim eulogized his father for nearly an hour, reading from the Koran and the Bible and sometimes speaking in Arabic and translating back into English. His theme was based on a sermon his brother had given the previous Sunday: "Dancing with Broken Bones." "My father danced with broken bones," he said gravely and often throughout his brilliant and impassioned "performance." At the end of the service, the black candle was extinguished and we proceeded to the cave for a final farewell.

The television crew was waiting for us. On arrival we assembled in the "lounge area," where Linda lit a white candle that symbolized reconciliation, forgiveness, and transcendence. Sadly, I noticed that the cave had already been ransacked and trashed. Broken liquor bottles were strewn about, and Cowboy's possessions had been pilfered. News about his death had spread throughout the streets, and "crack heads have moved in," reported Dr. Ralph. A few prayers were offered, along with remembrances of Cowboy. I offered the final prayer, concluding with the words, "Cowboy is no longer dancing with broken bones." I prayed silently that his soul had found peace, for secretly I agreed with Ibrahim. After the service Dwight went back to Ohio, his daughter went to Chicago, and Ibrahim went to his inner-city mosque. Linda and I, with friends who were in attendance at the service, went for a glass of wine and commiserated about the joys of having known Cowboy.

Cowboy is gone, but his story is alive and well, its lessons providing a map of the human condition. They show that the American institution of slavery and our societal history of racism are relevant in the twenty-first century. The evil of hatred and potential for cruelty that seem all too much a part of our humanity are shown to have had a fracturing impact on this man's mind and soul. They demonstrate the injurious consequences of poverty as well. On the other hand, they revealed Cowboy's creativity and love of life. He demonstrated a remarkable sense of resilience and inner strength. Perhaps most important of all, the lessons of Cowboy's story declare the redemptive power of love and illuminate the healing and transforming impact of "mindful presence" in the lives of the most vulnerable among us.

In gratitude for the care he received and for the attention of the students who became his friends, Cowboy left his body to the medical school so that even after death he might continue to teach the next generation of doctors. All I can do at this point is to hope and pray that, like Mrs. Angel, Cowboy will find rest, real rest, and peace, real peace. And that his narrative, along with those reflected in the other stories in *Dancing with Broken Bones*, will be heard and honored so that the legacy of John Treeo will be expunged, forever expunged.

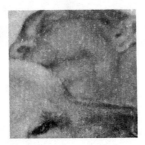